LIFE WITH CLARA

~ One Caregiver's Journey

MICHELE BERTAMINI

ISBN: 1453698213
ISBN-13: 9781453698211

Being in the group & sharing laughter (& empathy & support) for caregiver stories.

Most of us have observed either in real life or on television two older men meeting for the first time with a bit of awkwardness. Once it is discovered that they both are veterans, an instant rapport appears. No matter how different their lives are or their backgrounds, there is a commonality between them. Someone that may stumble across these two men minutes after their initial meeting could easily assume they have been friends for years by the ease of their conversation. These men that just met could share stories and experiences that they may have not even shared with their own family members. I have never served in the military or have fought a war, but I have experienced a similar phenomenon because of my role as a caregiver. I could be feeling a bit out of place at one of my husband's work functions but the moment I would find a fellow caregiver, an instant rapport appears. We now had a common ground. As a result, I could candidly speak of the range of emotions that I've experienced as a caregiver without fear of being judged. To try to have that same conversation with someone that never had to step into that role, there are too many things you have to try to explain. If you talk about your frustrations, it is interpreted as whining. Often a conversation with a non-caregiver about the rigors of being a caregiver, results in the non caregiver offering sympathies to you for a role they wonder if they are capable of fulfilling. That same conversation with a fellow caregiver, often results in laughter as you swap your 'war stories.'

Through my own experience, I learned things about myself that at times made me feel proud and other times ashamed. I used to think that anyone could be a caregiver, it was just a matter of stepping up to the plate when needed, but I'm not so sure anymore. You do not have to be a superwoman

i

to be a caregiver, but you do have to be willing to put portions of your own life on hold. At times I could do that cheerfully, other times with resentment. The funny thing is, I never liked the scary rides at the amusement park, and the most dreaded to me was the rollercoaster. Those few times I was coaxed into getting onto the rollercoaster, I would have to keep telling myself it would be over in a couple of minutes. Yet, here I was in the role of a full time caregiver, daily riding a rollercoaster of emotions with no way of knowing how long it would last. Some days I felt braver than others.

After years of taking care of our own place and primarily my husband looking after his mother's house, we starting talking about finding a place where we could all live together. My parents had purchased several acres of land and offered a piece of the land to us. My husband talked to his mother, explaining how difficult it was caring for two homes and two lawns and told her of our idea to build a house with an in-law apartment for her. Clara, my mother-in-law, was always eager to please her children, and agreed to this plan. When she moved in, she really just needed help getting groceries. My mother-in-law never learned to drive, yet still she was mostly self-sufficient. After the first five years, it was obvious her health was beginning to deteriorate, but she had refused to go to the doctors for the previous thirty years. Getting her to agree to go to a doctor would not be easy.

Clara loved to read, especially looking through the gossip magazines, and as her vision failed, she missed that. When I suggested that I take her to an ophthalmologist so she could read again, she reluctantly agreed. The day of her appointment she was so nervous that she didn't sleep all night. Little did I know what we were in for that day. The doctor was completely rattled and became unglued as he examined her eyes, which heightened Clara's nervousness. She was unable to see even the largest E on the eye chart, and the doctor could not believe how the back of her eye looked. Her retina was filled with so much blood and was continuing to bleed. He kept saying in a hyper tone, "Oh my God, oh my God." At this point, I was a bit rattled myself. I was completely floored when he asked Clara if she was diabetic and she admitted that she thought so. Both her mother and brother died of complications from diabetes, and I learned that day that Clara suspected that she had developed diabetes about ten years before, but was too frightened to go to the doctor for treatment. She had never uttered a word of this to us.

The eye doctor insisted we see a retina specialist that day and finally, Clara's fear of poor health was greater than her fear of seeing another doctor. Off we were to her emergency visit with the specialist. This doctor remained calm as he was examining Clara's eyes, but bluntly told her there was nothing he could do until she got her diabetes under control, and recommended an internist. On the way home, I asked Clara if she would let me take her to this internist and she agreed. At this point she was so scared; I think she would have agreed to anything. When I called the office, they did not have any openings for weeks for a new patient. I pleaded as I explained Clara's situation and I was told they would see what they could do. I was fearful that if I didn't get her to the doctor immediately, she would lose her courage and change her mind. Within hours, the doctor himself called to find out first-hand what Clara's situation was. After explaining what was said by the ophthalmologist and retina specialist he agreed that Clara needed to be seen immediately, and offered to meet us at his office on Sunday morning since there were no appointments available during regular business hours. Once there, he discovered that diabetes was only one of several significant health problems Clara had. Clara was close to fainting when the doctor told her he would have to take some blood for testing, she was so afraid of needles. Once this can of worms was opened, there was no turning back. Each visit resulted in more tests, procedures and referrals to other specialists.

In less than one year's time, I had taken Clara to more doctor appointments than if she would have gone once a year for a checkup the previous thirty years. As I learned Clara's family history and her own history, Clara would defer the responsibility to me to explain her history, symptoms and all of the medications she was now on. When it came time for Clara to start giving herself insulin injections she plainly told the doctor, "Michele can do that." I was grateful when the doctor referred the both of us to a nurse at our local hospital for lessons and this nurse demanded that Clara attend the session too. In my eyes, this nurse was awesome; she had dealt with the likes of Clara before. The nurse firmly and authoritatively told Clara she was not leaving until she learned how to give herself insulin injections. Inside I was cheering, because I did not want the stress of being the sole person responsible for giving her insulin. Clara resisted, but the nurse refused to take 'no' for an answer. Then the nurse informed me I had to give myself a practice shot so I would know how it felt, and then my attitude changed. Now internally I was nervous, but acted calm. I knew I could not expect Clara to do something I was unwilling to do, but I was not prepared for this! Clara finally submitted and gave herself a practice shot of saline solution, and then announced, "That wasn't bad at all!" and we all laughed. Personally I thought my self injection hurt, so I was quite pleased with Clara's response.

It was not possible for Clara to fill the syringes with the insulin because by now her condition was somewhere between legally and completely blind. I would fill the syringes; put the morning dosage on the top shelf of the refrigerator and the evening dosage on the bottom shelf. I took over more of Clara's meal preparation, since she had sent me to attend her scheduled visit with the nutritionist alone. At this point, I viewed myself more as a good daughter-in-law that was helping in the care of my mother-in-law, but not as a caregiver.

Chapter One

THE JOURNEY BEGINS

Describe

All of that changed on October 22, 1997, when I was thrown into the
role of full time caregiver and it felt like my life was turned upside down. Just
two weeks prior to that day, I had undergone outpatient surgery and was just
starting to feel recovered myself. It was a beautiful October day. My two sons,
Mike and Zack, had finished their homework and went outside to play ball. I
decided to take a quick nap before starting dinner. That's when I heard Clara
yelling for help. She fell and broke her arm which left her almost immobile.
As if a broken bone wasn't bad enough, she broke her arm right about where
it meets the shoulder. A cast was not possible so a sling was put on and it was
stressed that she had to keep that arm completely immobile. It was her right
arm and she was right handed.

As we got back home that night from the emergency room, Clara was filled
with fear, mainly that she would move her arm without meaning too. Clara's
eyesight had already put certain limitations on what she felt she could do,
and now she sat paralyzed with fear to even move. I was embarrassed when
Clara asked me to undress her and put her pajamas on, but my compassion for
her outweighed my embarrassment. I was ever so careful as I slipped off her
clothes, put her pj's on, then helped her into bed. The next morning, I was
over early to help her back out of bed and to her sofa. I tested her sugar level
as I had been doing regularly and then got her syringe of insulin out of the

refrigerator. Clara said she needed both hands to give herself the injection; one hand to grab a fleshy part of her belly, and the other hand the give the injection. Since she only had use of one hand, Clara said I would have to give the injection. I have to admit, the thought of it made me very nervous and I'm not normally a nervous person. Flashbacks of the session with the nurse during the injection lessons came to mind and I visualized the nurse standing over me like she had with Clara insisting that I give the injection. I also remembered that my injection hurt, and my biggest fear was hurting Clara. I was still having a hard time each morning poking her finger tip to get a drop of blood for the monitor to test her sugar level; I would apologize profusely each time. Now I had to add an injection to my guilt. I took a deep breath, gently grabbed a fatty piece of her belly and gave the injection. When finished I sighed with relief and announced, "It's done." Ever so sweetly, Clara said, "You have a gentle touch, I didn't even feel it." I wasn't sure if she was being truthful or not, but it gave me the confidence I needed for the evening shot and took a bit of the guilt away as to whether I was hurting her. That morning is when I realized my life took a drastic turn. Clara felt comfortable holding her cup of coffee and sipping it, but was afraid to feed herself. Again, it was a bit awkward to feed my mother-in-law like a toddler, but compassion was a good motivator to get me beyond myself. After feeding her and cleaning up the dishes, I went back to my portion of the house, but left the door open so I could easily hear Clara if she needed to yell for me.

Not much time had passed when I heard Clara yell, "Michele" at the top of her lungs. I scurried over as quickly as I could to hear the announcement, "I need to go to the toilet and I need you to get me up." Clara provided little assistance as I literally put my arms around her and picked her up. I escorted her to the bathroom and she asked me to pull her pants and underwear down. It seemed like each task was getting worse. I puttered around her apartment, doing some light dusting waiting for her to finish in the bathroom so I could help her back to her sofa. When I heard her call my name, I wasn't alarmed, until I found her still sitting on the toilet. I guess I didn't have a clue at this point because I asked her if she needed something, i.e. toilet paper etc. She said, "I can't reach, I need you to wipe my butt." Okay, there weren't any lessons for this one! My voice said, "Sure, no problem" but my head said, 'Gross, it stinks in here and that is disgusting.' I tried to imagine back to when my sons were very young and I was on butt wiping detail but as I leaned over Clara to wipe her, I thought for sure I was going to vomit. Old lady poop is nothing like I remember a three year olds poop smelling. I finished or so I thought, when Clara said, "Wipe it again." This time I kept chanting in my head, 'You can wash you hands in a minute, that's what soap is for;' over and over. I flushed the toilet still feeling ready to hurl, washed my own hands, then helped Clara up and pulled her panties and pants back up, and got her back to the sofa. She then asked what I was going to serve for lunch. Food was not foremost on my mind, but the bathroom incident was over and it was time to get back to the day and lunch was just a couple of hours away. Up to this day, I would typically eat two meals a day, but now I found myself thinking about food all of the time, planning Clara's diabetic meals and dinner for my own family. Before long I was eating three meals a day, and gained ten pounds the first month.

The next day wasn't as bad giving Clara her insulin injection but she had not bathed for two days and it was becoming noticeable. I knew what I needed to do, but I had never washed another adult before this. My main concern was for Clara's dignity, so I tried to act as nonchalantly as I could having to completely undress Clara, then help her into the tub; inside though I was dying of embarrassment. I'm a pretty modest person, I don't even like changing my clothes in front of my husband, and now I'm taking a washcloth to my mother's-in-law most private body parts. Never did I imagine this when we first came up with the idea of her moving in with us! Taking care of Clara was part of our plan, even though I didn't think it would come to this, it was what she needed. So here I am at thirty-seven years old washing my mother-in-law, thinking this is what my skin will look like when I am seventy-three years old, and it was an unpleasant look into the future! After her shower, I dried her off, helped her to her bed, where she sat as I put lotion and powder on her before dressing her. Oddly enough, I felt a closeness to Clara at that moment as if this experience bonded our relationship stronger, but not enough to make the experience of bathing her a joyful one. I even used some scented lotion and took several minutes massaging her feet and lower legs. Clara was so appreciative. I thought of how long she had been divorced, over thirty years and raising four children on her own. I felt sad thinking of how lonely her life must have been especially as her children grew older and moved out. I thought I would do something special for her every day. At this point I figured the worst was over, I had wiped her butt, showered her, and I still survived. This woman deserved to be taken care of. It wasn't long before I wondered if it was a caregiver that first uttered the expression, 'Ignorance is bliss.' The worst was yet to come and there was no way to prepare for it, so I was glad that I had never even imagined it.

The medication to help manage Clara's pain from her broken arm caused her to become constipated. At first, that seemed like good news for me since I was the only other female in the house so had been the resident butt wiper. Clara was starting to get up on her own and go to the bathroom by herself, and even trying to wipe herself using her good arm. I started giving Clara a stool softener to help things along, but after more than a week without moving her bowels, Clara was quite uncomfortable. That is when the call came, one that I jokingly named, "the call from hell." When I answered the phone, Clara said, "I had an accident, come over right away." I was at first naïve regarding what she meant, but reality quickly smacked me in the face when I opened the door leading to Clara's apartment. The smell was overwhelmingly nauseating and the sight was horrifying. Accident hardly described what had happened there. Clara was sitting in her reclining chair with a housecoat on, which confused me momentarily because I had not put it on her. I had my hand over my mouth and nose and I noticed there was dried waste all over Clara's legs and she said she felt weak. Well, to be honest, I wasn't feeling that strong myself!!! Once the stool softener kicked in, it did so with a vengeance. It all started while she was sitting in her reclining chair. She was tired of getting up for all the "false alarms" of when she had unsuccessfully gone to the bathroom. By the time she realized it was the real thing and stood up, poop was running down her pajama bottom leg onto the carpet. There was a trail of poop on the carpet leading to the bathroom. Clara still was having a bit of a hard time pulling her pants down with the use of only one arm, so when she reached the bathroom, she balanced herself in front of the sink while trying to pull her pants down.

As she leaned over, diarrhea actually shot out on the bathroom door. As she tried to rotate herself to get to the toilet, the same thing happened on the wall and the shower curtain. Now if you think reading about this is disgusting, it hardly compares to the actual experience. Her butt was already covered in poop, so when she finally sat down on the toilet, that created another mess. Clara was embarrassed and tried to clean herself up at the sink, but this was beyond anything a sink washing could handle. With her poor eyesight, she did not realize how much waste was still on her body. She left her soiled pajama bottoms and underwear on the bathroom floor and made her way back into the bedroom to get out a housecoat. When she sat at the edge of the bed on top of the comforter to get dressed, she got poop on that as well. She made her way back to her reclining chair and stepped in the diarrhea that was already on the carpet from her trip to the bathroom, and tracked it back out pressing it into the carpet. This is what I walked into and had no idea where to even begin. I told Clara that I was going to have to shower her, but I would clean up her bathroom first, and I hoped that she did not have to go any more. When I went back to the bathroom to clean it, I swear it looked as though a sprinkler had been set up in her bathroom that sprayed poop everywhere but the ceiling. To this day, it was the vilest thing I have ever encountered. I started with the dry heaves, but looked at the toilet and thought, 'there isn't even a place to throw up.' Desperately, I prayed, I begged for God to help me. I knew I could handle cleaning up baby poop, so I prayed for God to help this to smell like baby poop so I could do what needed to be done. The moment I finished my prayer and opened my eyes to this horrible sight, I started with the dry heaves again. So I hurried and closed my eyes and said, "God, I need a rush on this prayer!!" When I opened my eyes this time, the sight was still vile, but the dry heaves stopped. The smell was unpleasant, but not as bad. For the next two and a half hours I was cleaning up poop and did not have one more dry heave. No one will ever be able to convince me that I did not receive Divine help that day. Although the job of cleaning up Clara after she had soiled herself was something that repeated itself over the years more times than I can even remember, the first time was the worst, and I doubt I will ever forget that day. That dreadful day, after everything was cleaned up, I took some of Clara's Country

Apple scented lotion and put it on her legs and arms. After that, and even to this day, when I smell Country Apple scented lotion, it turns my stomach. My idealistic bubble of wanting to do something extra nice for Clara burst. Now it was about just trying to do everything that needed to be done.

It didn't happen right away, but in time my enthusiasm started to fade and I was hit with the stark realization that there is no retirement plan with this job. The only way out of this role would be to place her in a nursing home or when she died. It didn't make me feel very good about myself, thinking about either option. I admit, occasionally I would fantasize about Clara being in a nursing home, so that my two sons could become my main priority again, being able to establish my own schedule, and not revolving it around Clara's needs. Then images would flash in my mind's eye, things I had seen from visiting other patients at nursing homes, and I knew I would never actually be able to follow through on that. At times it was a nice fantasy to mentally escape to. Then there was the other option, her death. It's not a good feeling when you realize that your life would be much easier by someone else's life coming to an end. Even thinking about it would make me feel ashamed of myself and guilty.

Some time later, after Clara had healed from her broken arm, we were going out one evening as a family and Clara was going with us. My youngest son, Zack went over to see if she was ready for him to escort her to the car. He was around twelve years old at the time, and he casually walked back to our portion of the house. So I asked him why he wasn't helping his grandmother to the car and he said, "I don't think she is going out with us, she is taking a nap on the floor." My eyes met my husband's and we both took off running, but everything seemed like it was in slow motion. Clara was making slight jerking movements, but was unconscious. I thought she had a stroke. Andy, ran back to use our phone to call 911 for an ambulance. He never came back. I stooped over Clara, holding her hand, talking to her gently, telling her everything was going to be alright. I realized I did not want her to die, I hated seeing her this way, and it made me feel a little better about myself. I had to wonder if she was going to be a vegetable like I had seen other stroke victims become. That made me continue to reassure her, because I didn't know if she could hear me, if she was scared or if she even knew what was going on. It was quite a helpless feeling. It wasn't long before the paramedics arrived, and I handed them a typed list I kept of Clara's conditions and medications. I told them I thought she had a stroke but as soon as they saw on the list she was diabetic, they tested her sugar level. It was twenty-nine; she was in a diabetic coma. That sounded even worse to me but they said they could give her a shot they called a spike and to my disbelief, in less than one minute, she was coming around. They asked if I had orange juice and I quickly got a glass. Clara's speech was slurred but she was conscious. They helped her drink the orange juice and within three minutes her speech was normal and she was back to her old self. I had tested her sugar about two hours prior to this and everything was fine so I was completely baffled as to how this could happen. Then Clara revealed she didn't really like the dinner that I made her. She was getting tired of eating healthy, so she threw it away. I had already given her the scheduled insulin shot when I took over her dinner, but since she didn't eat, it brought her level down dangerously low. My sister-in-law, Maria who lives next door had come over to see if we needed help. After the emergency crew left, I asked Maria if she could stay with Clara for a moment. I went over to my side of the house to give Andy an update. Then I asked him why he never came back and he said he really thought his mother was dying and he couldn't bear to stand there and watch her die. I asked him if he thought that, why he left me to handle it and he said because he knew I could. I couldn't even be annoyed with him because I could handle it. However, the thought of my own mother laying there, (even though she is in great health), it took on a different dimension for me. As much as I loved Clara, I could detach myself to a point when I needed to do what had to be done, but I'm not sure I could have done that with my own mother. So it was easy to excuse Andy's absence during this crisis. Although I also could not have left her side, I realize everyone has their own way of dealing with things.

After that day, I was sure to keep that typed list I had about Clara's conditions and medications very current. I had an old prescription bottle that I used a garbage bag twisted tie to attach to the wire refrigerator shelf. I would roll up the paper and tuck it in the bottle. That way everyone in the house always knew where to find it. Later we asked Zack why in the world he would think his aged old grandmother would take a nap on the floor as he first reported to us. He said that we, meaning his parents, lay on the floor all the time to watch TV and figured that is what she was doing. That's when I realized, that even though I viewed myself as young and Clara as old, in Zack's mind we were both old without much distinction! I didn't have a scare like that again for several months.

When I would go over in the morning to start Clara's care for the day, she would already be sitting in her recliner with the TV on. One morning when I went over everything was still. I panicked that maybe she died in her sleep. Then I thought what a peaceful way that would be to die. From there I wondered if she did die, what would I do? I figured that I would dial 911. Now I had a plan of action, so I cautiously walked into her bedroom. She was lying very still on her side and her back was facing me, I could not see any movement and I just couldn't tell if she was breathing. My thoughts were all over the place, what if she didn't sleep well and finally got to sleep and here I am waking her up. What if she was in a diabetic coma and I was wasting time thinking when I could be saving her life. What if she was already dead, should I change from my pajamas before dialing 911? A complete nervousness came over me that made me feel physically shaky. With that, Clara cleared her throat and I felt like I jumped a mile, which startled her. I explained that she had overslept and I was checking on her to be sure she was okay. I skipped the part of all the scenarios that had been going through my head. It was actually a relief that she was alive and okay. As the years passed, on those rare days that Clara was not in her recliner when I came over in the morning, and I found her still in bed, my heart would beat a little faster, but I didn't have conflicting thoughts. Secretly, in my heart, I would hope that she was dead. I knew Clara wouldn't continue on forever, and I would worry that she would die a long, slow, painful death. My hope was that one night she would peacefully go to bed and not wake up. As I would stand there looking at Clara, wondering if today was the day, she would cough or clear or throat and I would think, 'Nope, not today.' On those days, I would feel like the most selfish person in the world because in my heart I knew my only motive was not that I wanted Clara to die peacefully, I wanted Clara to die to give me peacefulness. How did I get to this place? Those days were seldom, but happened just the same.

One day, Clara could not completely close the foot rest on her reclining chair, which meant she was not able to get out of the chair. Since she was getting up to use the bathroom, that meant another "accident." After cleaning her up, I inspected the chair and the foot rest was broken, it would not close completely. Off we were to the Lazy Boy Furniture store to find another chair that afternoon so Clara could test them out. She wasn't thrilled to miss her afternoon stories, but I insisted. Clara did not have the arm strength to use the lever to put the chair in the reclining position, and wasn't comfortable leaning back in the chair to get it in reclining mode, so that was something I would do for her. Getting out of the chair on her own was a priority, so I made sure she found a chair that was comfortable and that she could put the foot rest down and get out of. We drove home with the chair tied in and hanging out of the trunk of my car. I wasn't taking a chance that she would get stuck in her old chair again. She ended up spending so much time in her new recliner; I would call it her "Lazy Girl" chair.

Chapter Two

AUTHORITY OVERLOAD

Since I was the one that went to the dietician and the main one to take her to all doctor's appointments, I felt responsible for Clara's health and without realizing it, I took on the role of the boss. Especially when it came to her diet, I was the food police. On most Saturday's, Clara went out with her daughter to get something to eat, and sometimes stop at the store. It wasn't unusual for me to find some food item the next day that Clara was forbidden to have. When I would ask Clara about it she would act like she didn't know how it got there. At times, I would call her daughter and she said she had questioned her mother if it was something she was allowed to have and Clara would tell her that 'Michele said it was okay.' If it wasn't that she brought wrong foods home with her, she ate them while she was out. I could always tell by either her sugar levels being off, or her ankles and feet being extremely swollen or the bathroom "accidents." From the years of neglecting her diabetes, her kidneys were failing and we already knew dialysis was not far away. I would become so frustrated and angry because I felt like all the work I did the previous week was for nothing. It wasn't unusual for me to have to make Clara one meal at one time to keep with the eating schedule she wanted, then to make another meal for my family to eat when my husband got home from work so we could eat as a family. Clara didn't like most of the food that my family enjoyed, or they liked things that she could not have because of being on a sodium and sugar restricted diet. We mostly ate boneless/skinless chicken breast; Clara wanted more beef. My sons liked buttered pasta as a side dish, Clara hated that and wanted potatoes. My husband's preference was rice, so on most weekdays I made three different side dishes, and I won't even get into everyone liking different vegetables! So after putting that extra effort forth all week long, then seeing Clara's feet looking like balloons, I would well up with anger.

Once a month I would go to a local marina to reconcile their checkbook. I like doing that sort of thing and I really liked the owners of the marina, a husband and wife. I became friends with the wife, and we would talk about our families while I was there. She told me about her own mother, that had since died, who had similar health problems as Clara. At times she would tear up remembering how her mother would plead with her when she visited for a drink, and she would remind her mother that the doctor had her on a very restricted fluid intake. She would comment that if she knew how close her mother was to dying, she would have just given her the drink of water or whatever she wanted. Over the years of going to the marina, she would often express regret that she only could think about preserving her mother's life by following the doctor's orders exactly, and didn't think about her mother just enjoying her final days. When she would tell me these things, I would feel bad for her, but the message I think she was really trying to tell me went over my head. I still continued in my role of food police, being the boss of Clara's diet, after all, it was for her own good.

On another occasion, I was at a cookout with some other friends that I had not seen in some time. I was catching up with an old friend Shirley, when she told me her mother had recently died and I was sorry I had not known earlier. She proceeded to tell me about the day her mother died and how that day had some happy memories for her. Her mother's health had been failing and they knew she wouldn't be around much longer, so they made her favorite meal. Shirley went on to relate how delighted her mother was and how much she enjoyed that meal, and later that night fell asleep and never woke up. Shirley felt good about her mother dying peacefully. In my mind, I could understand giving her a meal that medically would not be considered good for her, she was down to her last days, and as it ended up, her last day. To me, I could not consider doing that for Clara. That would compromise her deteriorating health even more. In my heart I felt I was doing right by Clara and there was no other way.

For Clara, a woman that never really thought about healthy eating, just eating what she enjoyed, in retrospect I imagine I was obnoxious at times. I can only imagine how she waited for Saturday, to go out to eat without my oversight, to actually pick up a salt shaker and put it on her food, or order a bowl of forbidden soup. Each Sunday morning as I saw those swollen feet and ankles, I would feel I was the only one taking her health problems seriously. I could only see her diet from one viewpoint. As a result Clara became quite clever. We would often have our friends and our son's friends over to our house on Saturday for dinner and dessert. With Clara being out most Saturday afternoons with her daughter, it was easier to have company not having to take care of her too. During the week Clara would ask what I was planning on making. At first I would feel bad talking about foods that she wasn't allowed to have, so I would act like I wasn't sure, but Clara would push the subject. I would normally be excited about a new dish that I wanted to try making, or maybe a new dessert that I thought up on my own so it wasn't hard to get the menu out of me. I would ask her opinion and Clara would seem so happy to be a part of the meal planning. I would even tell her that I felt bad talking about foods that she couldn't have and she would say it didn't bother her. Once Saturday arrived and I was busy with my guests, I could hear Clara coming in her apartment and after some time I would run over to check on her. She would ask me how the evening was going and if they liked my new dessert. I was tickled that she took such an interest. Most of our friends know Clara, so one or two might wander over to her apartment to visit with her for a few minutes, and Clara would be delighted. What I didn't know is that when they would visit, Clara would scam them for dessert. Since she already asked me if my guests liked my new dessert, she knew that I had already served dessert. She would tell one of her visitors that I had promised her a piece of that chocolate cake that I made, but I forgot to bring it over. She would ask them if they would sneak over and get a piece for her, but not to say anything to me because she didn't want me to feel bad for forgetting. They knew Clara had serious health problems but figured she was telling the truth since she asked for the dessert by name. I typically served buffet style, so when I would see my dinner guest come back over from their visit with Clara and get some dessert, I figured they were getting seconds for themselves. If the evening would go on for some time, I would ask my husband to go over and check on his mother. She would ask for her nightly cup of hot tea and he would come back and say she asked for a piece of cake with her tea. I would remind him how bad that would be and he would say, "Can she have just a sliver?"

Looking back it is funny to me that he would ask me permission to give his own mother a piece of cake, but I was the self appointed boss of her food and he respected my self appointed authority. When I would take her tea over, I would take a sliver of cake with me, reminding her that she really should not have it, but for a special treat it would be okay. She would thank me so appreciatively and I never knew she had already wolfed down a full slice of cake. The next morning her sugar reading would be out of whack, and I would be trying to figure out how it happened, because one little sliver of cake should not have affected her that much. Other times, it would result in another "accident" and I would say no more of that dessert, but again it was hard to imagine that one sliver could cause such damage. A few times, Clara would have her "accident" while my dinner guests were still at my house. That would annoy me that I had to leave my own company to go over and shower her and clean up the mess. In my mind I was convinced it was because her daughter let her eat something bad for her when they were out earlier and I would resent that I was the one dealing with the consequences. I didn't realize it was mainly due to my own friends that had given her food from my own kitchen that caused the problem. It was actually a couple of years until I discovered it.

My oldest son, Mike had graduated from high school and we had a big cookout celebration at our house. We had about one hundred guests coming, and I did just about all of the cooking for it myself and I did not want to worry about taking care of Clara that day. By now, since Clara's kidneys were failing, she had little strength and when she went out she used a wheelchair. I called my sister-in-law and asked her if she could take care of her mother that day and she agreed that she would even wheel her mother outside to the cookout and

I would not have to worry about her. Since it was my first child graduating, I was quite excited and each day I probably bored Clara with the details, from the moon bounce we rented for the younger children coming to the canopy tents that would be set up, and of course Clara asked about the menu. It was a beautiful day and I was glad Clara could enjoy it. I was glad I did not have the added pressure of caring for her. That is the day I discovered Clara's food scam. As I was checking to see what food items had to be replenished, one of our guests asked if there were any baked beans left. I told her I had just put out a fresh, hot tray from the oven so her timing was perfect. She replied, "Oh, it's not for me, it's for Clara." I went right into food boss mode and said, "She's not allowed to have baked beans!" She apologized saying she didn't know, that Clara specifically asked her for baked beans. I thanked her for her help but was fuming that her own daughter was not doing her job. So I marched right over to her daughter, and told her that her mother was trying to get someone to get her baked beans. She looked at me and said, "She isn't allowed to have them?" I was in disbelief at that question and told her they were so full of sodium and with her failing kidneys she would end up with congestive heart failure from the fluid backing up around her heart. Her daughter said, "Mom said you said it was okay, she said you said for today it was okay for her to have hot dogs, baked beans, and that spicy macaroni salad you make." I looked at her wondering how she could not know those were the three highest sodium containing dishes I had. She apologized for giving her mother the wrong foods, I said what was done was done and it was a special occasion. I was telling one of my close friends that I was frustrated that the one day I didn't want to worry about Clara, I still had too because no one else seems to realize how important her diet is to her health. Then my friend said she felt terrible because Clara told her that I had promised she could have some baked beans but I must have forgotten with all that was going on, so she volunteered to get them. I wondered at that point how many helping of beans Clara had! So I went over to tell Clara she was busted and found her eating a piece of cake. I asked how in the world she got the cake, and another guest spoke up and said that Clara said I was supposed to get it for her but most have forgotten so she got it for her. That's when I realized why Clara was always so interested in knowing what my menu was, so she could ask different people to get her stuff she wasn't supposed to have. I told Clara she was slick and she just laughed. Later on I was telling some other friends about how my mother-in-law was slick as a fox and about her food scam. I ended up with five different confessions and that is when I learned that for the past couple of years each time I had dinner guests, at least one of them was taking some dessert over to her without my knowledge because Clara insisted they didn't bother me about it. She would even ask them to wait and take the plate and fork back so I wouldn't have to worry about it. They didn't realize they were being asked to hide the evidence! I had to laugh at how often I was outfoxed by this old lady. Of course the food she ate at the graduation party was over the top, and the next day I paid the price with lots of "accidents." I was physically exhausted from all of the work that went into the graduation party and felt low on patience, but she had to be cleaned up.

Sure enough, it wasn't that long before Clara was in the hospital with congestive heart failure. That just reinforced my thinking that keeping her on the prescribed diet was essential. Some time after that, her granddaughter, who was around twelve years old, was visiting for the day. I could hear a lot of yelling going back and forth and then my niece appeared in my part of the house asking, "Aunt Michele, can Grand mom have this?" She was holding up a big lollipop. I praised her for checking and told her that Grand mom could not have that. She replied, "I told Grand mom, but she keeps yelling at me to give it to her." I was so mad at Clara for yelling at her twelve year old grand-daughter for a lollipop. I marched right over, and with her lack of vision she didn't even realize that her granddaughter had left. She was still fussing at her for the candy. Normally, I could never raise my voice to Clara, I would feel certain things on the inside, but tried to show her the respect her age deserved. This day I was stern as I told her that I could not believe she was yelling at her granddaughter when she was trying to do the right thing by her. Clara seemed embarrassed that I knew what was going on. I then announced that I was retiring as her food police, that I was sick and tired of doing the extra work to keep her healthy for her to sneak around and undermine my efforts. I continued that I was tired of being the only one worried about keeping her healthy and I guess in dramatic fashion I told her to go ahead and eat the lollipop, she could eat five if she wanted to, I didn't care. My little tantrum seemed to take Clara aback and she said she didn't want the lollipop and she was sorry. I basically said too little too late and that I was retired and she could eat what she wanted. Clara apologized and said for me to continue feeding her healthy foods. In retrospect, I think her plea was because she felt like she hurt my feelings, not because she wanted more of the doctor approved foods. Little did I know at that moment it was the best thing that I could have done.

At first it bothered my conscience that I was falling down on my job as a caretaker. Finally, the conversations that I had from the marina owner expressing her regrets that her mother was deprived of the little joy she had in life before her death, and Shirley's conversation about her mother before she passed started to sink in. I was working so hard to keep Clara alive for as long as possible, I lost sight that the quality of life along the way is important too. As I reflected back on the four or so years that I strictly enforced her diet, I wondered if Clara was able to enjoy any of the meals I worked so hard to make for her. Clara wasn't a big sweet eater, so that wasn't the problem. Since she was in end stage renal (kidney) failure, she was supposed to have a limited amount of fluid and a very low sodium diet. When I would steam vegetables, I would even have to estimate how much water the vegetables absorbed and deduct that from her allotted fluid for the day. There were days she would ask for another bottle of water and I would have said she had her limit for the day and I would always feel bad. Now that stress was off of me.

Chapter Three

DIALYSIS-A NEW CAN
OF WORMS OPENED

It finally got to the point that Clara had to begin receiving kidney dialysis as she had become weaker and weaker. With her frail condition, she needed to begin as an inpatient in the hospital so she could be closely monitored. While in the hospital, Clara was unable to get out of the hospital bed without a lot of assistance. She was pretty much blind and was overwhelmed by the buttons for the television and to call the nurse. As a result, even if she had to go to the bathroom, she would wait until someone would come to her room, so she had a number of "accidents" in the hospital. When it happened at home, it was a matter of picking up the phone next to her Lazy Girl chair and calling me. Now at the hospital, quite some time would pass before an aide or nurse would come in for Clara to ask for help. Her butt became quite chapped and some special cream was ordered to soothe her skin back there. When either I or one of her two daughters would visit, she would ask us to rub some cream on her butt. We all came to call it her "butt cream." She probably had the equivalent of a baby having diaper rash, so I could understand why she would ask, but it didn't make the job any more pleasant. After Clara's broken arm healed, she was never able to reach behind her back with it, and now she was so weak with the heart failure from the fluid overload. She improved and we were happy to leave the "butt cream" at the hospital when we brought her home. Later that first day home, when I went over to check on Clara, she asked me to rub some butt cream on her. I told her I was sorry, that I thought she was all better, and I didn't pack it up with her belongings from the hospital. She said not to worry, she asked the nurse to put a fresh tube in her bag of belongings. Yes, outfoxed again by an old lady! It ended up being a very long day, and around 10:00 p.m. I told my husband I was going upstairs to take a nice, long bath. I wasn't in the tub two minutes when he knocked at the door. My voice wasn't pleasant when I asked him what he wanted and he said, "I'm sorry, my mother needs you." I got out of the tub with a rotten attitude, got dressed feeling sorry for myself and angry that Andy couldn't take care of his mother. As I flung open the bathroom door, he was apologizing all over the place, saying he heard his mother calling my name and he went over to see what she needed and she was in the bathroom saying, "Don't come in I'm not dressed, get Michele." My anger quickly faded and now I'm rushing over picturing her lying on the floor hurt. When I got to her bathroom she was sitting on the toilet with the tube of butt cream in her hand and said, "Michele, would you rub some of this on my butt?" I stood there thinking she was addicted to this stinkin' butt cream and that the person that invented it should be arrested and jailed. What do I do? I put on a latex glove, applied the butt cream and thought if any one dares buy another tube of this stuff, well let's just say no jury would convict me. I helped her back to her chair, and told her I was going to take a bath and her son would be over in a bit to help her to bed. It was always at those times she would thank me so sweetly that I would feel bad for allowing myself to get so frustrated. When I was going back to get in the tub, Andy asked what was wrong. I just started laughing and said she was having butt cream withdrawal. He started apologizing again saying he would have never gotten me out of the tub if he knew that is what she wanted, but it was okay. There were bigger things to worry about.

Dialysis opened a whole new can of worms. When it was determined that Clara would begin dialysis, I privately asked her doctor how long she thought she would live on dialysis. She explained with all of Clara's health problems, the hope was she would live up to two years. That was staggering to hear. It also gave me renewed enthusiasm for caring for Clara. This woman was down to her last two years of life, certainly I could tough it out and make her life as pleasant as possible. I had already scouted around a few dialysis treatment centers and found one about twenty minutes away from our house where the staff was really nice. Since she required treatment three times a week, which required three trips over, and three trips back. We divided up her transportation between me, my husband and her two daughters. In time, my husband's work schedule did not allow him to take his shift and it fell back on me. Eventually, her daughter that lives about a mile from us was only able to pick Clara up after treatment one time a week. So on Monday's and Friday's, I would take her and bring her home. On Wednesday, one of Clara's daughter's would take her, and the other one would bring her back home.

When Clara first started going there, she was in a wheelchair. The treatment would leave her even weaker, and once home, one of my sons would have to come outside to help me get her in the house without falling. Some times it seemed like her legs were wet noodles. To my amazement, after a couple of months, Clara had enough strength to use a walker. The first day Clara walked to the treatment area with her walker, all the patients and staff started clapping. Clara just beamed with excitement. Within six months she was walking without the walker, but would have to hold onto someone's arm for balance. Even her eye sight started to improve and she could see patterns in clothes.

Before she started receiving dialysis, you could stand in front of her and wave your arm and she couldn't see. Even with her improvement, the doctor said he doubted Clara would live more than two years on dialysis since she neglected her health for so long. Dialysis would last around three hours, and after she was settled in her treatment chair, I was not allowed to stay. I was grateful for that rule, because if not I think Clara would have expected me to stay to keep her company. I found a small portable CD player and started getting some CD's of artists she enjoyed. After getting her settled in her treatment chair, I would hook up her CD player, put the headphones on Clara and adjust the volume for her. Sometimes as I was leaving, she would start singing along and it was a pleasant way for me to leave her, in a good mood. Often when we arrived at dialysis at her appointment time, they were not ready for her. Usually problems arose on earlier treatment shifts which would make things run behind. Clara would get so aggravated when she had to wait, which always struck me funny because what else did she have to do? I'm a friendly and outgoing person, so I would get chatting with other patients that were waiting, or patients that had finished their treatment, but were waiting for a ride home. Clara's hearing wasn't that good, but I would try to draw her into the conversation to make her feel included, and she loved that. We became friendly with quite a number of patients. The only downside was the days we arrived and they were running on time. After I would get Clara situated, these older patients still expected me to sit and visit with them for a bit. Some were still in the treatment area and I would stop by for a brief hello on my way out, but the ones sitting in the waiting room were a bit harder to get away from. Sometimes, it would take me another half hour just to leave. There was one patient there named Martin, he was just in his early thirties. Martin was very kind hearted. Clara and I both felt so bad that such a young man had such serious health problems. He was usually finishing treatment as we were arriving, but would always stop and find out how Clara was doing. One miserable, rainy day when I was leaving, I noticed Martin standing at the bus stop across from the dialysis center. I stopped and asked where he was going, and he said to the light rail station. That was less than ten minutes away, and I could not leave in good conscience with him standing in the pouring rain without any rain protection. He was grateful for the ride and told me that each Friday he took the light rail into Baltimore City to stay with relatives for the weekend. Later that evening I told my husband what I had done and asked if he minded if on Friday's I would ride Martin to the light rail after dropping his mother off. Andy knows I like to be helpful, so he did not object. Martin seemed appreciative and took my kindness in the way that it was meant. Unfortunately, after some time one of the nurses asked me if Martin was my boyfriend. I was humiliated that someone that saw me a couple of times a week bringing my mother-in-law to dialysis would think I was using it as a place to pick up a man. After that I was not comfortable taking Martin to the light rail station, but also was too embarrassed to tell him why. On some Fridays when the weather was nice I would ask my oldest son Mike to take his Grandmother to treatment. That was always a welcome relief from the Martin problem. Even then, some days that same nurse would ask, "Did you see your boyfriend Martin today?" I could only hope she was kidding.

On most days after dropping Clara off for treatment I would be back home by 4:30 and I would start cooking dinner. On dialysis days Clara would eat a big lunch, and just a light snack afterwards, so I didn't have to worry about cooking for her those nights. This one day, my husband was out of town for work, and I wasn't really hungry, and I decided to make grilled cheese sandwiches for my boys and maybe a can of soup. Yes, the lazy mother's dinner. Mike said he wasn't in the mood for that and was going to run out and grab some fast food. He had his own car and his own money from his part time job, so I said to go ahead. Not fifteen minutes had passed when he called and said he was involved in an automobile accident. When I arrived it was a mess, the police officer was yelling at my son for driving reckless and for causing this accident. I was proud of how respectful my son was responding to this officer that was right in his face. As I walked over to intervene and find out exactly what happened, the officer started with an attitude towards me. I actually asked him to calm down so I could ask my son what happened and he said, "I'll tell you what happened" and started again with his reckless driving speech. I turned to my son and asked if he was hurt and he said he was. I was in disbelief at how this officer was acting and asked one of the paramedics that was standing nearby if he could help my son, which he did. It was quite a scene with a ·crowd gathered around. There was a woman standing nearby who asked if my son was okay so I asked her if she witnessed what happened. She went on to tell me that a middle aged woman had run a stop sign and ran into my son's car and that the woman accepted responsibility but the officer told her there was no way he believed that an eighteen year old male was not driving recklessly. I immediately went over to the woman that was pointed out to me, the one that ran the stop sign, introduced myself, and asked if she was okay. She started apologizing to me for hitting my son, she said I could be proud of my son because he had been berated by this police officer and he stayed respectful the entire time, even before I arrived. I asked her if she would come with me to speak to the officer again while the paramedics were strapping my son to a back board. The officer agreed to write in the report that my son did not accept responsibility for the accident but still had a nasty attitude. Between dealing with that and knowing that my son wasn't seriously injured, but injured just the same, my emotions were all over the place. As they loaded him up in the ambulance I told Mike I would follow right behind him. Then I realized the time, by now Clara had to be picked up from dialysis in half an hour. I told him I would be there as soon as I could. He was good about it, he understood our lives revolved around his grandmother's needs but I was so resentful that I had to put my mother-in-law ahead of my own son. I called ahead to dialysis and explained the situation and asked if they could have Clara's CD player and things packed up and her ready to walk out the door when I arrived and they were very accommodating. As I was getting Clara to the car I was telling her what happened and of course she expressed her concern for her grandson. As we were driving home she said, "I'm really in the mood for my cup of hot tea when we get home." In my mind, I had pictured pulling up to the house, swinging open the car door and having my younger son Zack help her in the house. I told her I really didn't have time; I was already much longer in getting to the hospital than I wanted. Clara said she understood but really was looking forward to her cup of hot tea. At that point, I could not think of the frustration she must have felt needing to depend on someone, all I could think is that she was being a self centered old lady that could only think of her own needs. Thank goodness for cell phones, so I could call home and ask Zack to put on the tea kettle so the water would be ready when we got home. I got to the hospital and Mike was doing fine without me, flirting with the nurses. I knew he really didn't need me there, but I needed me to be there. He was released and we went home, him feeling sore from the whiplash, me being angry and resentful towards my mother-in-law. Even though it all worked out, I was still angry at being put in the position that I had to choose. It was probably a good night for my husband to be out of town.

    After two years on dialysis, a new dialysis center opened just five minutes from our house. Yes, Clara was still alive. Clara had made such remarkable progress, it was obvious the doctor's initial estimate of her life expectancy was wrong, and we started making provisions to transfer her to the new location. On one hand it was the greatest of compliments to be told by medical personnel that Clara was living much longer than they ever anticipated because of the care I provided for her. On the other hand, some days that was a conflict of interest for me!! Clara wasn't thrilled about changing where she would receive her dialysis; she was used to going where she was. I kindly pointed out to her that while she only had a twenty minute ride over, I still had another twenty minute ride to get back home, that did not include having to come back after her treatment was over to pick her up and drive back home again. Clara said she did not want to change, but understood it would be selfish on her part not to. I decided that it would also be good for me since I had become attached to so many patients at the old center, and since that required so much of my time; I was not going to get involved with anyone at the new dialysis center. I was so excited the first time we went to the new center. We left the house, I got Clara weighed and set up in her treatment chair and I was back home in less than 20 minutes. With not knowing any of the other patients I didn't feel the need to stop and visit with anyone. Since it was a new center, they were not filled to capacity yet, so Clara's chair was always ready when we arrived. After being at the new center for just a week, when Clara and I walked in, the wife of one of the patient's was throwing a fit. She was cursing like a sailor at the staff, angry that her husband's treatment did not end on time. I put my head down to mind my own business and was trying to hurry Clara back to the treatment area, but Clara would take these baby steps and it seemed like it was taking forever to reach the treatment area. This woman kept asking me what I thought about the inconsiderate bunch here and I'm still trying to hurry Clara thinking I DON'T WANT TO GET INVOLVED. I was even tugging on Clara's arm a bit trying to hurry her, but I think Clara was intrigued by the commotion and was trying to figure out what was going on. This woman walked over to get me to join her in complaining, I just said that we were new here and I was sorry she was having a bad day. As we finally got in the treatment area, I told the nurse that we were in no way connected to the angry woman in the reception area. I didn't stop to think that they would know who this woman was since her husband was a patient; I was just so worried about getting off on the wrong foot with this new center. Each time we would arrive for Clara's treatment, this woman would be yelling and cursing about something. Since there was no avoiding her, I decided to break my own rule and try to befriend her. I found out that she worked at a nursing home. She arranged her schedule to go to work after her husband's dialysis, so she could pick him up and transport him home. Her loud complaining was because her husband had not finished on schedule and it was making her late for work. In time, it seemed like this woman, who I came to call Miss Betty, would wait for us to arrive. I would always try to calm her when she was agitated, and in time I learned a lot about Miss Betty. It became clear she had a hard exterior, but was a woman full of pain and love to give on the inside. She had a very difficult childhood, and there were many things about her adult life that wasn't that great either. Eventually, when we arrived, we never found her yelling, just sitting around talking with others in the reception area, and I would always have a quick visit with her after dropping Clara off. We ended up forming a friendship that surpassed the dialysis center. In time her husband died, I visited her at the funeral home and found out from her children that she spoke warmly of me. As Miss Betty's health has declined, I have visited her during hospital stays or extended nursing home stays. I try not to let too much time go by without keeping in touch. I was glad I broke my own rule with her since our friendship continues to this day.

Then there was my other experience that did not turn out well at all. For the first year, Clara was almost always assigned to the same treatment chair. There was a man that was always in the chair two seats down from Clara. He looked like he was around my age, maybe a few years older. Out of the corner of my eye I could see him watching us as I would get Clara situated. Clara was supposed to stand until the technician or nurse could come over to get her blood pressure. Most days, just the walk from the car to the treatment area would tire Clara out and she would get grumpy if she had to wait more than ten seconds to have her blood pressure taken. So it was easy for me to learn how to do it, so I could take Clara's standing blood pressure. Then she could sit down and get comfortable in her treatment chair. Each chair had its own TV, so I would turn on the channel Clara wanted, put her headset on, and adjust the volume. Then I would take her sitting blood pressure and usually by then one of the technicians or nurses came over to start Clara's treatment and I would leave. I could just feel this man watching me the entire time, but I dismissed it as boredom of his surroundings. However, I was still careful not to look his way or even say hello. I really did not want to give any wrong signals to him or to any of the nurses that were watching. One day this man was in the chair next to Clara, which was probably four or five feet away. As I finished with Clara, I just nodded my head towards him as to say hello, because it seemed rude not too. That was the extent of things for some time. Then one day Clara was seated on the opposite side of the treatment area and this man was seated near the doorway by the exit. As I was walking towards the doorway I could feel him looking at me and I gave my head nod and he put his hand on his heart and was patting it. I wasn't sure what to make of that, and I kept on walking, but he just looked at me and patted over his heart. There was not a nurse in sight, and I wondered if he was having chest pains and here I am walking right out past him. So I went over and asked him if he was okay and he said he had gone to a funeral that morning for a friend of his. I expressed my sympathy for him and told him I noticed he had a tie on and now I understood why. He said for me he would wear a tie everyday if I wanted. Oh, good Lord, what did I do to deserve this? It's not much of a confidence booster attracting a sick man surrounded by elderly patients! I again told him I was sorry about his friend and left. On my way home I had to laugh at myself. That night I was telling my husband about my stupidity and he said, "Michele, you are at a center filled with health care professionals, and you think you are the one he is going to tell he has chest pains too!" I like be helpful, and sometimes I don't use balance. Once I became Clara's full time caregiver, it seemed to make me think I had to stop and help everyone that I thought needed help. It's a nice quality in some ways, and one that leads to problems in another, especially since I wasn't always balanced with it. After that day at dialysis, I tried to go back to acting like I didn't see him. Once again he was situated in the chair by the door and as I was leaving he took his index finger and made a motion like you do when you want someone to come over. Not learning my lesson, I walked over and asked if he was okay. He said I looked very nice that day. Something about this man made me feel dirty and degraded the way he would speak, even though he did not say anything that I would consider crude. I kindly thanked him and continued on my way. About a week later when Clara and I arrived he was in the reception area. This was the first time we arrived that he was not already in the treatment area and as Clara and I approached the door at her usual snail's pace, this man was at the door opening it. He held the door in such a way that I would have to brush up against him to get through with Clara. I said, "I appreciate you being such a gentleman, but it is easier for me to get Clara through the door by myself." He stood to the side, but as we got inside the doorway, he said in a low, disgusting voice, "Ha, ha, ha, I'm no gentleman." He said each word slow and deliberate. It really gave me the creeps and I could feel my heart racing in fear. I'm trying to hurry Clara along like I used to when Miss Betty was throwing her fit and Clara yelled, "Slow down, stop rushing me." He just stood there looking me up and down. When we got to the scale to get Clara's weight, she asked me who the man was that was at the door. I told her it was the man I told her before that tries to get me to come over to his chair. She said that she could not hear what he said but his tone of voice gave her the creeps. As we were walking back to the treatment area, I was telling her what he said and told her he made me feel scared. Clara was so sweet, she said just to stay with her for awhile, until I was sure he was back in the treatment area and out of the reception area. When I left, I called my sister Kathy. I had told her about this man's strange antics before, but related how he was waiting at the door and how he made me feel. Then I told her I knew I was being silly but that I really felt scared when I left. She gave me a strong lecture and told me many rape victims had bad feelings about someone they knew, ignored those feelings as silly then later were victims of that same man. I told her that this man was sickly and he probably just wanted attention. By the time she was done with me, this man now felt like a real threat to me. When we got home from dialysis that evening, it was already getting dark and no one else was home. Our home is in a wooded area and I was paranoid looking all around.

Even though I can normally talk to my husband about anything, I was embarrassed to talk to him about this man. I had already told him about the first encounter, and he correctly pointed out how foolish I was to think this man was calling me over for medical help. So I figured he would really think I was being silly about the entire thing. The following Monday morning, I drove over to my girlfriend's house so I could walk with her and her husband for exercise. We would walk very early before having to start my day with Clara. As we were walking, I was relating how I was dreading going to dialysis that afternoon because of this man and I related my experience. Her husband asked what my husband thought of it and I told him that I was too embarrassed to tell him and why. He told me that this man sounded like a real threat and I really needed to tell Andy about it. He also told me it was important for me to alert the staff at dialysis of my concern. First my sister, now my girlfriend's husband is telling me not to ignore my gut reaction. It was hard to believe this man was a real problem but it was also hard to ignore that he could be. Andy was already at work and I had to take Clara to dialysis but I promised I would tell Andy as soon as he got home from work. After getting Clara set up in the treatment area, I asked to speak with the head nurse. I told her my three experiences with this man and she said she knew exactly what I was talking about. She told me he often makes her feel uncomfortable. Then she said what worried her is that this man works at the Motor Vehicle Administration and she worried he would run her car tags and find out her home address. Now this didn't feel like my imagination running away anymore. The head nurse said she could talk to him on my behalf and I told her I felt it was important for me to deal with it directly. At this point, I felt intimidated when I walked into the dialysis center, and I wanted to get my control back. I just wanted to alert her to my plans.

That night, I knew I had to keep my promise to tell Andy. I asked him if he remembered the man that patted his chest and he laughed and said yes. I told him about the next time he used his finger to call me over and he stopped laughing. As I got to my third encounter, he was on the edge of his seat. Rather than feeling like I was going to be blamed for creating this problem, Andy was ready to go to battle for me. At this point I just told him what happened, not even my reaction to it and Andy said this guy sounded like a real problem and potential threat. As I told him how scared I was all weekend, he couldn't believe I didn't tell him sooner. He told me not to worry, that he would take care of the matter immediately. I thanked him, but told him I felt it was essential for me to at least try to handle it first, because I felt this man took some control from me and replaced it with fear. I needed to get my control back. Andy reluctantly agreed that I could handle it first. I wondered if any other caregiver found herself in this mess! The next treatment day Clara's daughter took her, so I had until Friday to practice my speech. I told Clara on the way what the plan was. So after getting her situated, I walked over to this man's chair. He was smiling flirtatiously and I began my practiced speech in a stern and authoritative voice, "Sir, I'm not sure how you could have gotten the wrong impression of me, but let me assure you, I do not appreciate the tone and manner in which you have been speaking with me." With that he interrupted me and said, "I don't know what you are talking about, you always come over to my chair, you are the one that comes over to see me!" Oh, I realized how I had been set up, that is why he was always so discreet in his hand gestures and waiting for no one else to be around. I was furious at this point, but he interrupted my speech and threw me off for a moment. I thought if I don't take control of this situation right now, I will never get it back. So I interrupted him and said, "Sir, you know what I am speaking about and I am here to tell you that I do not appreciate how you have been talking to me, my husband does not appreciate how you have been talking to me, and my grown sons do not appreciate how you have been talking to me." Again he says, "I don't know what you are talking about." I continued, "Yes you do, I'm telling you - it is stopping right now." With that I turned on my heel and left. My heart was beating a mile a minute but I felt like I got my control back. After that when I would walk into the treatment area with Clara, I could see him turn his head the other way. Some months later I did not see him anymore and was told he received a kidney transplant and the entire staff was glad to see his treatment end.

About a year after my last conversation with this man, I was walking down the aisle of a home improvement store and I could see this man walking down the aisle towards me. My initial reaction was panic, my heart started racing. I hurried and turned my cart around and went into the next aisle. Then I thought how silly it was to let this man scare me, and I turned my cart back around and went back to get the items I needed. This man was still in the aisle, and I stood there confident and sure, at least on the outside. When he walked by me, he spit in the back of my head. It rattled me, but I laughed out loud as if it didn't and said, "What a big baby." Afterwards, I thought I should have screamed that I was being assaulted to see how he responded to the store staff coming to my assistance. What a mess, from just trying to show human kindness to another. That was my only bad experience from this dialysis center, the staff was very nice.

I became friendly with the nurses and technicians, but it was not the same burden that keeping tabs on so many patients had become at the other center. When I would run into the staff at the mall or grocery store, we would stand and chat for some time. Often they would express the respect they had for me for the care I gave to Clara. I had never received any commendation from Clara's other children for the care I gave their mother, so that meant a lot.

Taking Clara to and from dialysis two times a week didn't seem like a big deal anymore. I still had to arrange my day around her, but it was better. Since Clara was getting stronger, I would often make her lunch in the morning and put it in the refrigerator, so she could get up and get it out herself. After dialysis, she always wanted a bowl of soup. She loved the soup from a restaurant that was only about fifteen minutes from our house. I would often drop her off, go pick up her soup order then go about my day until it was time to pick her back up. Once she was home I would warm the soup up and make her nightly cup of hot tea. Providing her meals was no longer the ordeal it was when I was carefully cooking each meal according to her dietary restrictions. I would consider Wednesday my day off because after I went over in the morning to take care of her, I would not have to worry about her again until the evening. By now Clara's dialysis time was moved up to noon, so on Wednesday her one daughter would come and take her to breakfast, then to dialysis, and the other daughter would pick her up on her way home from work. At first I would still have to be available when she got home to give her a light meal and her hot tea. In time I asked her daughter to take care of that which she did, so until 11:00 p.m. when Clara was ready to go to bed, I was off duty.

After being involved in several car accidents (none were my fault) I was having trouble healing because of the physical demands Clara put on me with helping lift her up. I arranged for a physical therapist to come to the house for Clara to help strengthen Clara's arms and legs. I would go out to receive physical therapy or other treatments for myself. At bedtime Clara could sit on the edge of her bed, but needed me to pick up her legs and put them into bed. I asked my husband if he could help with that and that became his duty. Clara was a stickler for her schedule. She wanted to be put to bed at 11:00 p.m., not a minute before and if we were not there at 11:00 p.m. exactly, by 11:01 p.m. the phone would be ringing. Clara could look sound asleep in her lazy girl chair but the moment the 11:00 p.m. news came on she would pop up and be ready to go to bed. On days my husband was out of town for work, sometimes I was tired and wanted to go to bed earlier, but Clara would be resistant to going to bed early. For the most part, she was sweet and easy to get along with, but she was a creature of habit and it would rattle her to try to change her schedule. On those nights I would ask my son Zack to put her to bed, and he usually didn't pay strict attention to the clock, but knew his grandmother would call by 11:01 p.m.

My problems resulting from the car accidents I was in were getting worse. I even went under some painful procedures to help. It would only take one incident of Clara having trouble getting out of her chair with no one else being home to help and I had to help lift her up that would undo all the progress I made. I finally sat down with Clara, and as kindly yet firmly as I could explained that I wanted to take care of her and never wanted her to go to a nursing home. I told her I had observed when the physical therapist was coming, she made quite a bit of improvement, but after the therapist released her from her care, she would refuse to do any of the exercises, most of which were done while sitting in her chair. Clara just listened. I told her in order for her to stay living with us I required three things from her; that she be able to get up out of her reclining chair by herself without assistance, be able to get out of my car without me pulling her up, and to be able to get off of the toilet by herself. I asked Clara if she felt that was unreasonable and she said it was not. Then I added that if she could not do any of those three things, I would no longer be able to care for her because my health was being compromised. Before I finished my sentence Clara was marching her legs in place while sitting, one of the exercises she previously refused to do. I knew Clara trying to do more for herself was good for her, and I really needed it. After that, there were many times she said she could not get up, and I would remind her that I could not help her and she would try a bit harder and be successful. There were other times that she wasn't feeling her best and she refused to try again. At first I would end up helping her, then feeling frustrated and resentful because it would cause muscle spasms in my neck and back, often resulting in a migraine with vomiting.

One day I was helping her in the car and somehow she sat on the ledge of the car frame instead of the seat. I was in disbelief that she missed the seat. There was just no way she could ever get up from sitting so low to the ground, and of course no one was home and I said a cuss word at her. I have always worked hard not to use foul language, I thought the words many times, but always wanted to set a good example for my family and just didn't say them. Here I have my eighty-one year old mother-in-law sitting on the edge of the car saying she was going to fall out on the driveway, scared to death, and I pick this day to mutter my frustration by saying, "Oh SHIT!! I can't believe you missed the seat." Then I felt like a big bully. I told her not to fall off the ledge that we would work it out together. I had her wrap her arms around my neck and I wrapped my arms around her waist and on the count of three I picked her up. I wanted to pick her up to the seat but she wanted to stand back up and then try sitting again. So I got her standing up, but she is now so out of sorts, her legs were buckling under her. With authority I said, "Clara, stand straight, strengthen your legs" and she did. Our way of getting her into the car was to back her up until her calves felt the frame of the car, then she would sit on the seat, and I would swing her legs into the car. It was a good system. We worked together and got her in, by now I was drenched with perspiration and embarrassed that I cussed at Clara. As I got in the car and turned the air conditioner on, I apologized to Clara for saying a bad word to her out of frustration and she sweetly said, "I didn't even hear it." Her hearing was bad, but not that bad, those were the things she would say that would endear me to her. Off we were to dialysis and we got laughing about something else. After that day, she would try to grab her pants leg with her hand to help lift her own legs into the car, she was trying.

Chapter Four

HELP ARRIVES JUST IN TIME

One thing that I will always be grateful for is our local Department of Aging. When Clara's health first started to decline, it was suggested to me to put her name on a waiting list for future help if needed. Around the time Clara started dialysis, her name came up on the list. A nurse came to the house to assess Clara's needs and it was determined she qualified for help through their program. It was a big disappointment when I realized that only moved Clara's name onto a second list, help was not immediately available. There were many names ahead of Clara's that were also approved for assistance. It was another year before I received a phone call asking if Clara was still in need of help. I was eager for any help that could be provided. The nurse came back to reassess Clara's needs, and determined she qualified for a home health aide that could come three days a week to bathe Clara and do some light housekeeping. Out of everything I did for Clara, giving her a shower was what I hated the most. With the aide coming three times a week, I asked Clara's daughter if she could shower her on Saturday when they got back from their afternoon outing. That only left three days that Clara would need to wash up at the sink. I did a happy dance of excitement at the thought of retiring from shower detail! Things were actually getting better. At first it seemed like as soon as Clara would become comfortable with her home health aide, they would quit or change their hours. Since they came on Clara's dialysis days, we did not have a lot of flexibility on what time they could come. Sometimes, there would be several weeks between health aides coming. After getting a break from bathing Clara, I would dread it even more going back to it. In time we were assigned a kind hearted, hard working home health aide named Alice. Alice would always go the extra mile. In time, she and Clara developed a friendship and Alice always had a listening ear for me if I had concerns about Clara I wanted to share. Both Clara and I developed a deep fondness for Alice.

Vacation time proved to be a challenge for my family. Clara's other children worked full time and did not always want to use their vacation time to care for their mother during that week. Sometimes they were able to work things out, other times I would have to make the arrangements for Clara's care. The difficulty was being able to find someone that was willing to start their day with Clara at 8:00 a.m. and end their day at 11:00 p.m., with lots of stuff in between, including transportation to and from dialysis. Since Clara was not always stable on her feet, people were afraid she would fall so did not feel comfortable taking on the responsibility of getting her to dialysis. The Department of Aging provided transportation, but you had to be able to walk from your door to the van without assistance. At least I did not have to worry about finding someone to bath her; the aide would still come for that. Planning time away never was easy.

One time, my brother and sister-in-law, Tom and Barb, invited us to go to New York City with a group of friends to see a Broadway show. We were to leave Friday afternoon and return Sunday night. Andy and I were excited about the trip, and I was also excited at the thought of having an entire weekend off from Clara. This time her daughter was able to take Clara to her home to care for her. My oldest son, Mike was on Spring break and flew down to Georgia to visit a buddy. Zack was going to stay with friends. We could actually go away worry free and just enjoy the weekend. We drove over to pick up Tom and Barb and before we were out of their driveway my cell phone rang. It was Mike asking me how our health insurance worked out of state because he thought he broke his wrist. I gave him instructions on going to the emergency room. At first Andy was getting aggravated by the apparent change in our weekend, but I calmly told him there was no reason to change our plans. Mike was five states away, there was nothing we could really do for him, and that he was with friends and a broken wrist was not the end of the world. My preference would be to go with him to the emergency room, but since that wasn't possible we continued on with our New York trip. I still felt really good about getting away. On the way, after several unsuccessful attempts to reach Mike by cell phone, I started to worry. So I called one of the mother's whose son also went on this trip, and asked if she had heard anything. She had not, but promised to call her son and call me right back. When she called me back she said things were not good. It appeared that Mike broke his left wrist and right elbow and was in a good amount of pain. She said she told her son to be sure to have Mike call his mother. The tone of our carefree weekend was changing. When I hung up the phone I started to cry and say, "If he has to go to the bathroom, he can't even wipe his own butt!" Wonder why that was the first thing that came to mind? By now we were only an hour away from our New York hotel, and we were the transportation for Tom and Barb too. At first I wanted to turn around and go back home to Maryland, but Mike was still in Georgia. We had passed Newark International Airport and my husband said if needed, we would fly back home. I only cried for maybe 20 seconds, but it was enough to change the entire tone of the trip. Once I spoke with Mike, he sounded good, but said he just wanted to come home. I tried to make arrangements with the airlines, unfortunately a strike was looming and there were no available seats until the next morning. I worked off and on through the night and was able to get Mike a return ticket home. Tom and Barb kindly agreed to cut their trip short and drive home with us Saturday night after the show we already had tickets for, since no one else in our group had room in their cars for them. I then called my other brother Jim, who lives next door to me to explain the situation. Mike's plane would land before we could get home, so Jim quickly agreed to go to the airport to pick him up. I knew his wife, Maria, would smother and mother Mike, just the way I would want to if I was there. Before we left New York, Barb started with a migraine headache accompanied by severe nausea. Similar feelings of having to choose one person over another person that I dearly loved resurfaced. It is such a no win situation I felt in, it left my entire body tense and anxious. I was also tired from being up the night before trying to make

Mike's travel arrangements, and then sight-seeing all day long. Barb was in the worst condition and that poor girl climbed into our back seat armed with a trash bag in the event she vomited. I wondered if she was feeling about me the way I felt about Clara the night of Mike's car accident when I had to send him off to the hospital by himself while I went to pick Clara up at dialysis. We got home around 4:30 a.m., and Mike was sound asleep in his bed with gauze and ace bandages wrapped around both arms. To me he looked pathetic. I knew Clara would be home in just a matter of hours, and I did not get the break I so desperately wanted and needed.

First thing Monday morning after taking care of Clara, I was able to find a highly recommended orthopedic surgeon to take Mike to. Due to his swelling, they did not put casts on Mike at the emergency room in Georgia. He was instructed to see a doctor as soon as he got home. Being considered an emergency patient that was being squeezed into an already fully booked schedule, I felt completely nervy asking if they could work with me around my mother's-in-law dialysis schedule. Fortunately, the doctor's secretary was very understanding and worked Mike in right after we dropped Clara off to dialysis.

Before Clara, Mike and I left, Mike managed to put on swim trucks, climb into the bathtub holding his arms up so the gauze would not get wet, and I helped bathe him. I kept teasing him calling him "Grand mom" and he teased back saying I'd better be careful, or he would ask for some butt cream. He had not shaved his face while he was away, so that duty was left to me. Of course with his age, I would leave the bathroom for him to dry off and get dressed. From the bathroom, I answered the phone to find out that Clara had an "accident" and needed my help. I went over to take care of that mess and finish getting Clara ready for dialysis and the three of us were off. It ended up that Mike had broken both of his wrists that required casts. His elbow was not broken, and the injury there did not require a cast. We were able to get to dialysis with both of Mike's arms in casts just as Clara finished. Once home, Zack helped me get his grandmother inside, who was ready for her hot tea and her evening snack. As I went to my stove to put the water on, that is when Mike announced he was hungry. I knew the care Mike needed was temporary, so it wasn't as overwhelming as it sometimes felt like with Clara. Mentally, I so needed that break from Clara that weekend. Technically, I did get a break from her, but it did not feel like it since I was worn out from trying to get my son home and myself home to him.

Life goes on and now I had to figure out how to get Mike to all of his college classes since he could not drive. The dialysis center was great about adjusting Clara's time to work around Mike's classes. I was the home health aide for bathing Mike in his swim trunks. I would start with taping plastic bags over his casts, and fortunately I have a large shower stall in my bathroom. Since Mike is a half of foot taller than me, I would stand on a step stool in the shower, while he held his arms high above his head, I would wash his hair. He would yell that the water was running in his eyes and as I would wipe the water away, he would complain that I was wiping his eyes the wrong way. I was ready to place both him and his grandmother in a nursing home! Mike healed ahead of schedule, and we were both glad when the casts came off two weeks early. At first, going back to just having Clara to care for seemed easier. Soon, summer was here and we were off to the beach for our annual week long trip with my side of the family. Arrangements for Clara were made and I must admit, getting up each day without thinking about her care was wonderful. I noticed by the end of our trip, a feeling of dread came over me at the idea of returning home. The first morning back, Clara had an "accident." While cleaning up poop was never my favorite activity, it was especially annoying this day. Later that day my sister Kathy called to see how everything was back at home, and I was complaining about Clara's accident. Kathy said she had the perfect solution. The next time I had to clean Clara up, just have her sit on the toilet, and take the toilet brush down her butt crack and back up again. She said Clara would never have another "accident." Of course she was kidding, but the mental image was hysterical to me. There were times after that when I would be cleaning Clara up, I would get that mental image of using the toilet bowl brush, and I would have to fight back from laughing. Another time, Clara had made quite a mess, and I was on my hands and knees cleaning poop out from in between her toes. Unknown to me, Clara in her desire to help, picked up the wash cloth off the shower shelf and slapped it in between her legs to clean that area. To my horror, dirty water splashed on my face and in my mouth.

humor

As I looked up she was pulling the washcloth back out and I pleaded, "No, no, please, give me the washcloth!!!" My eyes felt as big as saucers and I could not believe what had just happened. I was trying to spit out whatever was in my mouth and wipe off my face without using my dirty hands! Once it was all done, and I thought of how it must have looked, I found it all funny. Later I was relating to my mother what happened, but she did not find the humor in it. Her protective mother instincts came out and expressed anger towards Clara. I told her that I try to help preserve Clara's dignity when she has her "accidents" no matter how I am feeling on the inside. My mother said, "I think in preserving Clara's dignity, you lost your own." I shrugged it off, but the next time I was cleaning out in between Clara's toes (with the washcloth far from her reach), I thought to myself, 'My mother is right, I have no dignity.' Then I thought of Kathy's suggestion with the toilet bowl brush, and some how, those two things made the job of cleaning up Clara's mess funny to me. Some time later I told my mother how her words actually provided humor to me when I needed it, and she did not even remember saying it. On one hand I felt that I wanted to protect Clara's dignity, but on the other hand my way of coping was to relate my experiences to family members or friends in a comical way.

Less than nine months after Mike broke both of his wrists, he sustained a serious shoulder injury while playing football. At first, the emergency room doctor thought he had dislocated his shoulder. After looking at the x-rays, he realized it was much more serious than that, and surgery would be required. It was a holiday weekend, and Mike was sent home with pain meds until we could follow up with an orthopedic surgeon. I found someone that specialized in the shoulder, and again was able to get an appointment that worked with Clara's dialysis schedule. We learned that Mike needed major surgery and would have up to a six month recovery time. His right shoulder injury prevented him from having use of that arm before surgery, and of course Mike is right handed. Insurance red tape prevented the surgery for ten days. We had been sent home with pain medication for Mike to take every four hours. The doctor said this was a painful injury and to give him the medicine every four hours before the pain got bad, and to be sure to take the medication with food. Of course, Clara still wanted everything done for her exactly on the schedule she like, no

humor as coping

flexibility there. So at 2 a.m., Mike's scheduled pain medicine time, I would ask Mike if he just wanted some crackers to take with his medicine. He really wanted mashed potatoes with gravy. Granted, he would accept instant mashed potatoes and jarred gravy warmed up, but even that seemed like too much effort in the middle of the night. After taking his pain meds, he would be back to sleep, but as the four hours were coming to an end, I could hear him groaning in his sleep in pain. At 6 a.m. he would be asking for Oodles of Noodles, and as he fell back to sleep, I would be back up at 8 a.m. to start my day with Clara. At 11:00 p.m. after Clara was put to bed my sink would be empty, by morning it was filled with pans, dishes and glasses.

The day of Mike's surgery fortunately fell on a non-dialysis day. I made arrangements with my mother and Maria to help care for Clara. After surgery Mike ran into complications, and we were at the hospital much longer than anticipated. He really needed to be admitted but our health insurance would not allow it. I was so glad Zack was home to put his grandmother to bed so I didn't have to try to figure that out. Andy and I did not get home until after midnight and Mike was in an incredible amount of pain. We had two sofas in our family room, Mike slept on one, and I slept on the other to care for him. I continued getting up every four hours to give Mike something to eat so he could take his pain meds. I could not get much rest even when Mike was sleeping because I could hear him moaning in his sleep. Zack was old enough to get up and ready for school on his own, but there was still Clara, there just never seemed to be a break from Clara. It seemed to me that her daughters never volunteered to do any more than their one day a week. That day getting Clara to dialysis seemed like it required the last little bit of energy I had left. The first week after Mike's surgery was the worst, and I was still on his bath detail.

Each year my husband takes our sons and my brothers on a 'guys only' ski trip, and that was fast approaching. We asked Mike's doctor if he could go to hang out with the guys, and the doctor said he had to be careful even playing cards, not to use that shoulder at all. I was nervous for Mike to leave but looking forward to the break. He was weaning himself off of the pain medication, and starting to do more for himself. I knew he would never expect the guys to do for him what he expected from me. I guess the lack of sleep for three weeks

• when care magnifies

never a break

took its toll on me, and I became sick. My husband offered to stay behind, but I shooed him and my two sons out the door. By now I was running a temperature averaging 102, and just wanted to stay in bed. Unfortunately, this weekend Clara's daughter was also away. Whether or not I wanted to take care of Clara, it still had to be done. I would set my alarm to wake me up when it was time to care for Clara, go back to bed and set my alarm for the next time. Each time the alarm would go off I would feel sorry for myself that I had the burden of taking care of Clara. I was angry that every one else could go off when they wanted, but I was always left holding the bag of responsibility, and it wasn't even my mother. In my mind that weekend, I was a practically a martyr. Each time I went over to Clara's it was with an attitude. When my husband would call home to check on me, I was sure to tell him just how rotten I felt. He felt bad that I was sick and still had to still take care of his mother. Good, that's how I wanted him to feel. Yes, being sick made me really ugly! My mother would call to try to help, and being the martyr I would not allow it. It would make me so mad that my family was the one always offering to help me care for Clara, and not Clara's family. I thought of all the times I had to take Clara to Johns Hopkins Hospital to see one specialist or another. They were such long days. Just getting her there was eventful. I would pull up to the entrance, help Clara out of the car, find a place to leave her propped up, run back to my car, go to the parking lot, then hurry back to where I left Clara, hoping she was still vertical. Then we would enter Johns Hopkins and hope Clara could make the long walk to the area she needed to be seen. Eventually I discovered the valet service at the hospital and took advantage of that. It made it so much easier pulling up to the curb, getting Clara out and not having to worry about the car. By now we had a wheelchair for Clara which helped quite a bit. I thought of all the surgical procedures she had done that mostly fell on me. Sometimes Andy would leave work and check in for a bit, but then leave to go back to work. Clara's daughter would come and do the same. One time after a surgical procedure they both came and left. In recovery Clara ran into complications, and there was talk of admitting her overnight. I was left there alone to deal with this crisis, and Clara was quite distraught. It ended up that Clara stabilized enough to be discharged and by now it was the height of rush hour traffic and it was snowing hard. Clara was given pain medicine to hold her over until she got home. They could not give her too much, or she would have been unable to walk once we got home. Now we were stuck in terrible traffic, moving only three city blocks in twenty-five minutes and I'm panicking that Clara's medi-cine was going to run out and she would be suffering and there was nothing I could do about it. The responsibility I would feel for Clara would become overwhelming, but it had to be done. By the time we got home, there were sev-eral inches of snow on the ground, Clara was quite weak and in pain. Although Andy is quite particular about the care of our yard, when I got home I drove the car across the front yard to Clara's door. Mike and Zack came out and helped their Grand mom inside. Even my grown sons had a struggle to get her inside and I thought, 'What if they were not home, what would I have done?' I prayed that I could get the car back to the driveway without getting stuck. Inside I thought I dared for Andy to say something to me about driving over his lawn. To me desperate times, desperate measures! It was snowing so hard, that in no time my tire tracts were filling in. That feeling of being in this with Clara all alone, despite the fact that she had her own children was a source of sadness and frustration for me. Of course, those feelings were exaggerated in that I did not have to do one hundred percent of everything myself without ever receiving help, but often I was left holding the bag of care for Clara. It just seemed to be expected, and seldom appreciated. That would create emotional turmoil for me, fighting feelings of resentment towards her own children. The ski weekend brought those feelings to the surface again. As I laid in bed feeling horrible, those were some of the memories that came flooding back. Although Clara would express concern for me, she still wanted her hot tea on schedule, to go to bed when she wanted, etc. The weekend came to an end, the guys returned, I was feeling a bit better, and Mike no longer required extra assistance from me.

My mother, cleverly trying to think of a way around me to help out, offered to take Clara out to lunch on Thursday. Clara enjoyed it so much that my mother would invite other friends to join them the following week. Clara came home in the best of moods, and on those days she would not need me to make her lunch, worry about her in the afternoon, and for dinner she would want a danish and a cup of hot tea. How easy was that?! Even one of her daughter's noticed how happy this made Clara, so my mother agreed to take Clara out every Thursday for lunch. Some times I felt guilty that my mother was doing my job, but she reasoned with me that it wasn't my job, I was just the one doing it and she was glad to help. I had another break that I was happy for.

Chapter Five

CLARA AND CARLY

My boys always wanted a dog. I had a dog growing up and loved him, but it was easy since all the responsibility fell on my mother. I could remember sometimes it was hard for my mother to find someone to care for the dog when we went on vacation. Every couple of years, the subject of getting a dog would come up and I always stood firm against it. With the boys getting older, my husband was weakening in his resolve to stand firm on our refusal to get a dog. The boys picked up on that, and knowing he was the weak link, would talk about their desire to get a dog when I wasn't around. Mike really wanted a Doberman, and Andy had seen a picture of a red Doberman and thought it was pretty. One day Andy brought home a magazine on Doberman's and I reminded him how difficult it was to get someone to care for his mother when we went on vacation, I didn't want to have to add finding someone to take care of a dog on top of it. Andy told Mike and Zack my reply. That was all the ammunition Mike needed, the son we would call, 'Attorney Mike' for his relentless techniques in badgering you until he got what he wanted. Mike played on my guilt, the guilt I felt because of the time I had to devote to caring for Clara that used to be devoted to them. I knew what he was doing, but it still made me feel bad. Then he waited a couple of days and came back and said now that he was getting older he wasn't home as much, which meant Zack often came home from school to an empty house if I was out involved in Clara's appointments. He argued what a difference a dog would make, a companion for Zack when I had to take care of their grandmother. I knew he was playing me, but guilt is a terrible motivator, and I agreed we could get a dog. I knew the promises they made of doing all the work were worthless, that it would fall on me. I did worry that Zack felt lonely or neglected at times because of the time I spent with Clara and the thought of getting a dog made me feel a bit less guilty. Before long we were driving home with a crying nine week old red Doberman that the boys named Carly. I held her like a baby in my arms trying to soothe her, wondering what had I done agreeing to this! Once word got out that we were getting a dog, some friends gave us some helpful advice on crate training and other techniques on having a puppy. We thought we were all ready, but were ill prepared for this puppy. Clara had some fond memories of dogs she had in the past as pets, and seemed to bond with our new puppy quickly. Carly did not like the crate, and rather than feeling secure in it as we were told she would, she would go in full panic.

When we would go out, after taking care of Clara, I would have to try to coax Carly into the crate. If I laid on the floor next to the crate, she would settle down but as soon as I would walk away she would become hysterical. When we would return home, we would have a mess. Carly would poop in her crate, something we were told dogs never did. Then in her hysterics to escape she would step in it and pieces of poop would be flung all over the crate, through the grates of the crate and on her. She was so hyper and relieved that we returned home, it was difficult to calm her down. Any poop in her paws would be tracked on the carpet. Once we opened the crate door, one of us would take her up to the tub to give her a bath, another one would take the crate outside to hose it out, one would clean up the area around the crate and paw prints, and one of us would go over and check on Clara. It got to the point that we tried to schedule our lives so someone was always home, which was not possible. Since Clara would often be home when we went out in the evening, I asked if the puppy could stay over with her in her apartment and she said no. She was worried if she had to get up to go to the bathroom she would trip over the dog. I could understand her fear of falling, but was frustrated that she could not do this one thing to help us out since the dog would always move out of her way when she was up.

When I was home during the day, Carly had so much love to give us that I quickly bonded with her. After several weeks of her hysterics when we would leave and return home, Andy said he thought we would have to get rid of her because she was doing too much damage to the house. In my mind I thought if that was the criteria for staying or going, that his mother should have been gone years before! I was smart enough not to say it, but told him I would check with the veterinarian for suggestions. The vet said Carly had separation anxiety and gave us some reference material to consult. I tried all the techniques, one by one, without any success. So Mike and I worked out an arrangement that when we went out as a family we always found a reason to take two cars. One of us would find an excuse to leave ahead of the rest of the family, get home and clean up the evidence from the dog before Andy got home so we could keep her. Whoever was left behind was to stall Andy to give the person home as much time as possible to clean up. I could not believe that my life now revolved around an old lady and a dog! It became evident that this crate training was never going to work for us and I took a big risk in going out one evening and leaving Carly free reign of the first floor. I didn't know if I would come home to our furniture being chewed up or something else destroyed. Knowing that Andy would have never agreed to let the dog loose unsupervised in the house, Mike and I continued our technique of one of us always beating Andy home. To my great surprise and relief, the first time home there was no damage, and no poop to clean up. She was still hyper and hysterical when we would get home, but we would take her outside and let her run out her energy. Of course, that didn't mean I didn't still come home sometimes to Clara having a poopy mess. At least now, I was back down to only having to clean up after one family member. Only after a month of successfully letting Carly free reign of the first floor, did I let my husband in on our secret. By then he had stopped talking about getting rid of the dog because he had bonded with her too. It was nice not having that pressure of one of us always having to beat him home. Each time I would go over to Clara's apartment to care for her, my new shadow, Carly would be right behind me. She would put her front paws on the arm of Clara's chair and give Clara a great big lick on her cheek. Clara would laugh with delight. A few times, Carly took advantage of Clara's limited vision to steal a few crackers from her. Clara would treat Carly as if she was her grandchild, laughing at her antics and sharing her food. It became our morning ritual that after taking care of Clara, I would give Clara a handful of Wheat Thin crackers and she would feed them to Carly one by one. Carly would take each cracker very gently and every morning Clara would say the same thing, "I can't even feel her teeth... good dog, you take food so gentle." Then when all of the crackers were eaten, Clara would say, "Where's my kiss?" With that Carly would jump up and give Clara a big wet kiss on the cheek and Clara would laugh. That was a nice part of my morning with Clara. Although my reign as the food police had ended, there were still some nights I would cook for Clara. I would put thought into what I made and tried to make something pleasant and mostly healthy. Especially since the food she ate from restaurants was usually high in sodium. Some of those nights Clara was the only one I was cooking for since we would have plans to eat out. After putting forth that effort, Clara would occasionally say, "I don't want that, feed it to the dog", I would be infuriated. I know she didn't mean to sound so ungrateful, but it was hard not to take it that way.

When Clara would be in the hospital from time to time, Carly would look all over the apartment for her and as soon as Clara would return home, the routine would continue. Even though things improved after we stopped putting Carly in the crate, it seemed like three hours was her limit with being left home alone. If we weren't home within that time frame, something of ours would be chewed up when we returned home. I asked Clara if I could just keep the door between our house and her apartment open while we were out, so if Carly felt stressed being alone she could come over to see her. Clara still refused. I continued to try some of the techniques I read to lessen Carly's anxiety, and eventually got to the point that she could be left for five hours. You can imagine when it did come time for us to go on vacation, it wasn't just a matter of having someone stop in and check on the dog. We actually had to pay someone to stay at our house during the day and spend the night. Since she was more anxious as a result of us being gone, the person could only leave her for a couple of hours each day.

I would always give Clara's daughters our vacation schedule at the beginning of the year so they would have plenty of notice, so that wasn't a worry, or so I thought. A young man that we had known for some time agreed to stay at our house the week we were away to care for the dog. He worked outside and said he would welcome the break of being out in the summer heat all day but he was not comfortable taking care of Clara too. I assured him that Clara would be at her daughter's house for the week, it would just be him and Carly, and we agreed upon a price. Two weeks before our vacation, I got a call from Clara's daughter that they were not going to be able to care for Clara; they decided to go on vacation the same time. I didn't know what to do and Andy was furious when I told him. He said we made arrangements for the care for his mother while we would be away, and they were it. If they wanted to change the arrangements, then it was up to them to make alternative plans. I told him in theory that sounds great, but the reality was they could get in their cars and leave. We could not get in our car and drive to the beach for the week leaving his mother to fend for herself. That was the reality of our situation. Now I had to figure out how Clara was going to get to and from dialysis, her meals for the week and her care. Fortunately, Alice was still her aide that would come to bathe Clara three days a week. That woman was a gem. She agreed she would come prior to dialysis and bathe Clara, feed her lunch, then take her to dialysis. I arranged for someone else to pick her up and bring her home. Then each day I had a different friend of mine bringing her food and checking on her. This was the vacation we took with my family, so they were not home either to help out. Having the young man staying at the house to care for our dog gave Clara confidence in the evening that she wasn't all alone. Once we returned home, Clara had nothing but complaints for the meals she received; they were not what she had in mind. Eye yi yi!! Clara had come accustomed to me revolving my life around her and her needs, and didn't like to accept anything less than that. By the following January, I again sent a letter to Clara's daughters, letting them know the dates we would be away and would need their help in caring for their mother. This year was more than usual, a four day weekend in April away for our anniversary, five days in May for a trip my husband won through his work, and then our annual week long beach trip in August. I received the letter back with notes next to the dates saying in April they could only help two days, May, one or two days, and in August they were available, but that was subject to change. From my perspective I wasn't asking too much and was frustrated by their response. My mother and sister-in-law Maria were always willing to volunteer to help me with Clara, but I felt like I should not have to depend on my family. When it came down to it, they were the ones that made it possible for us to get away for those extra trips, and I was very grateful for that. We had not heard anything about the August trip, but I was holding my breath based on what happened the year before.

By now, Mike was engaged, and his wedding was about a month after our beach vacation. His fiancée, Tanya, was going to join us for the weekend at the beach, and then we would have Mike with us for the rest of the week. We realized what a turning point we were in our lives, and were really looking forward to this vacation. Two weeks before our trip, I found out Clara's one daughter and husband at the last minute were able to book a trip to Italy. It amazed me how their vacation time again coincided with ours. The other daughter was going to be in town and she was going to care for her mother while we were gone. Since Tanya could only join us for the weekend, she came up to our house Friday night after work so we could get a very early start on Saturday to the beach. I explained to Clara that I would be coming over earlier than usual and that her daughter was going to come later in the morning to pick her up for the week. When I went over in the morning to care for Clara before leaving, I said my usual, "Good morning." She turned her head to look out the window. I thought maybe she didn't hear me so I repeated myself and she turned her head again. I could not believe what a baby she was being, not speaking to me because we were going away and leaving her. As I stood there in the kitchen in my disbelief at her behavior, looking at her in her Lazy Girl chair I realized she kept turning her head straight then to the left. Then I realized something was very wrong, it was as if her head was involuntarily turning back and forth. When I stood in front of her I knew, she had had a stroke. The first time when she went into a diabetic coma I incorrectly thought she had a stroke, but this time I was absolutely certain. She had a blank stare in her eye, and drool was coming out her mouth, her head kept turning back and forth and she made mild grunting noises. At that moment I thought all of my care, all of my hard work came down to this, Clara was now a vegetable. I remembered reading articles on stroke victims that they can hear you even if they cannot respond. I calmly told Clara it would be okay and that I would get her help although I was shaking on the inside. I used a tissue to wipe her drool away, and my heart just broke seeing this shell of a woman. This situation was pathetic. I told her I had to call for help, but I would be right back. I didn't want her to hear me calling 911 on her phone and hearing me describe her status, I thought it would be better to use my phone. When I walked through the door to my side of the house, Mike and Tanya were getting ready to head out to the beach. I explained what was going on and asked them to go and watch Grand mom while I called for help. I didn't know if she could fall out of her chair or not, and instructed them to talk gently and calmly to her. After calling for help, I informed my husband who was upstairs finishing packing his clothes for the trip, and then called her daughter. I went back over to Clara's, and Mike asked if they could still leave for the beach. At first his question took me aback, your Grandmother is sitting in the chair grunting and unable to move and you want to go to the beach? I thought for a moment, and realized whether he stayed or left, it would not change the fact that Clara was now a vegetable. I asked if he could stay until the ambulance came to help keep the dog out of the way, then he, Tanya and Zack could leave. He readily agreed. Once the paramedics arrived, they tested her sugar and the level was fine, which confirmed my belief it was a stroke. As they loaded her on the stretcher and got her in the ambulance, Clara's grunting got louder. Minutes later her daughter arrived, with the ambulance still sitting in my driveway, I was getting worried that she was in some sort of distress. I knocked on the back of the door of the ambulance and they said they were just trying to get an IV started. With Clara's condition from dialysis, getting IV's started was always a challenge. Clara was mumbling now, and didn't seem as vegetative. From my description on the phone and seeing Clara for herself, her daughter said, "She's not that bad." She was just moments earlier. Andy and I drove in one car, her daughter wanted to drive over in her own car, and we followed the ambulance to the hospital. By the time they got her settled in and allowed us back, Clara was back to looking vegetative. It was hard for Andy and his sister to witness. Clara was paralyzed on the right side, when the nurse picked up her arm it was as if it was dead. I secretly wondered if Clara was going to be one of those people that lived for years as a vegetable since her heart was strong. I knew I would not be able to completely pick Clara up to care for her as she would now need. The thought of her in a nursing home in that state made me sick to my stomach. Tests were run and it confirmed that she had a stroke. A neurologist was called in and treatment options were explained. A clot busting medicine could be given, but since she was already on blood thinners, she could bleed internally causing her death. Without this medicine, she would remain in a vegetative state the rest of her life. Even though I was the most involved in Clara's daily care, I felt it was important for me to yield to Andy and his sister, they should make the decision. They both agreed there was no choice and approved this medication to be given to their mother. There was only a small window of time that this medicine can be used following a stroke, and we were just about out of time. The doctor called the pharmacy to quickly get this medication down to the emergency room, and the nurse started the necessary preparations for Clara to receive this medicine. The doctor also ordered a blood test. The nurse inserted the needle to withdraw the blood and when she attached the tube to collect the blood, Andy noticed his mother scratching her head with her right hand, which moments earlier was completely lifeless. Apparently, the vacuum effect of this sealed tube for collecting her blood moved the blood clot and blood flow was returning to Clara's brain. Just then the clot busting medication arrived and the doctor halted its administration for a few moments to observe. Within minutes Clara was speaking, her speech was quite slurred, but her thoughts were coherent. Her paralysis was mostly gone, but she was more limited on her right side than before this stroke. She said she heard everything the paramedics were saying and they were annoying her because they were hurting her inserting the IV. We were all in disbelief. The doctor said Clara would be admitted to the hospital for several days. I knew I had even more work ahead of me once she was discharged and I was thinking that I really would like to relax on vacation before having to face that. How could I ask Andy if we could still go on vacation with his mother lying in the hospital hours after suffering a stroke? I excused myself so I could go get a cold drink, it was now five hours since I had awakened and had nothing to drink or eat. I needed to think. On my way to the cafeteria I was racking my brain as to how to approach the subject of our vacation without sounding like the most selfish person in the world. When I came back to the room, Clara was resting comfortable, and her daughter had gone to call home to inform her family as to her mother's status. Andy said to me, "I don't want to sound rude, but I still want to go on vacation." Ahh, my dilemma solved! I told him we knew that she would be getting care at the hospital, and with cell phones, we were only a phone call away, and less than three hours away at the beach. When his sister returned we told her we were going to head out soon for our vacation, and she had the same look I think I had when Mike first asked me if he could still go to the beach. Clara woke up and I made sure she understood what was going on and she did. She was in a great mood. We told her we were going to head out for the beach and she said to go and have a good time. On the way to the beach I would get calls here and there with questions about Clara's medication or history so I still felt connected to her care. I battled with feelings of guilt for still going on our trip. The next morning I called the hospital and Clara was in the intensive care unit. The nurse offered to take a phone over to Clara. It was unbelievable, Clara wasn't even slurring her speech anymore, her speech had returned to normal. As word spread of Clara's stroke to our friends, some went over to the hospital to check on Clara. None could believe how chipper she was. She needed to stay to receive some intensive physical therapy before returning home since the use of her right arm was still limited. Her daughter would go to work each day and then stop at the hospital on her way home and stay for hours. I know it had to be hard on her, but I thought of all the times I had that duty. I wasn't feeling mean spirited about it, but the reality was the bulk of the work was going to fall on me once she was discharged. By Thursday we still had two days of our vacation left, but by now I felt like I was being greedy. I told Andy that I just didn't feel good about staying any longer at the beach since we had not seen his mother in five days. He said it was getting hard on him too, so we cut our trip short and headed home. My sons stayed at the beach. We drove right to the hospital and Clara was delighted to see us. She asked why we came home early and we told her it was because of her and she laughed and said, "No really, why did you come home early?" I don't think she ever completely believed she was the reason we came home early, which perplexed me based on the care we regularly gave her. By now Clara had been moved to the rehabilitation section of the hospital.

The next day I met with her team; her nurses, therapists and social worker. They asked me what my expectations were. I told them I required three things from Clara; that she can get out of bed in the morning on her own, get out of her chair without assistance and to the bathroom unassisted. I then heard their report, Clara had significant loss of motor function on her right side from the stroke, but they were surprised that her left side was also affected. I kept my mouth shut because most of what was described to me was Clara's condition before the stroke. The team felt confident they could help her gain her strength and I knew the stronger Clara was when she returned home, the less wear and tear on my body. After our meeting, I went to Clara's room and her first question was, "When can I go home?" I told Clara she would need some more treatment, and reminded her that she needed to be able to get out of her lazy girl chair at home by herself. This floor kept Clara busy with differing types of therapies, and she was missing most of her stories in the afternoon, she was not happy. I reminded her that the more effort she put into physical therapy the quicker she could come home. I would only visit Clara for about an hour each day, I felt this was my time to get what I needed to get done before Clara's return home. Her daughter would come after work and stay until after visiting hours each evening, so I felt like my visit during the day was enough. Once her other daughter returned from Italy and learned of her mother's health crisis, she rushed to the hospital. Then she was back to work and limited in her time to visit. One day when I arrived for my daily visit, I walked by the nurse's station to go to Clara's room and noticed a large group of patients were sitting around a table. I continued down to Clara's room and it was empty. I went back to the nurse's station to find out if Clara was in therapy, and the nurse pointed to the table of patients. I didn't even see Clara when I had walked by before. The floor was hosting an ice cream social and Clara was in the midst of the patients chatting and laughing, it was nice to see. Clara seemed delighted that I was there. I noticed Clara's hair had been done and when I complimented her on it she told me a hairdresser actually came to the hospital and washed and set her hair. She was so tickled about that and asked if I had money to pay the girl, when I said yes she said, "Be sure to leave her a good tip." I thought back to the morning of our beach trip, looking into Clara's vacant eyes hearing her grunting, to now, a little over a week later, with a sparkle in her eye and communicating perfectly. The lady next to Clara asked, "Are you her daughter?" I answered, "No, I'm her daughter-in-law Michele, it is nice to meet you." Clara piped in, "But she is as good as any daughter you could ever hope for." She actually teared up when she said it, Clara didn't express much sentiment and her remarks deeply touched my heart. I thanked her and told her how delighted I was to see her doing so well. The ice cream arrived, so I told Clara I would come back later so as not to interrupt their ice cream social. On the way home I had tears in my eyes as I thought about Clara's kind words.

After a week in the rehabilitation section, Clara was making it loudly known she wanted to go home. I quietly did love not having her home. I met with her team again, and they felt confident with Clara continuing her exercises at home, she would continue to gain strength. I explained that I had arranged for Clara to have physical therapy at home in the past, and while the therapist would come, Clara would give one hundred ten percent knowing the quicker the progress, the quicker her release. However, she would never continue her exercises after being discharged from therapy. I expressed my concern that after she was discharged from their care, I was confident she would refuse to do any of the exercises, even the ones she could do sitting down. This team felt Clara had a renewed enthusiasm for getting better and they were confident she would continue her exercise program at home. By now I think I was pleading with them not to send her home just yet, saying she needed a few more days of therapy under her belt. Part of it I wanted a few more days too without being the primary one responsible for Clara. I was assured things would be fine and at that point I relented. I knew that sly fox Clara had tricked them into thinking she enjoyed her exercises and would continue with them at home. Sure enough, she was discharged later that day, and the next morning when I went over to do her exercise routine with her she said, "Not now, maybe later." As predicted, later never came. Clara came home in better condition than before her stroke, but in less than a month, without continuing the exercises, she was back to where she was before all of that therapy. I had to remind Clara again, physically it was too demanding on me to lift her out of the chair; she had to do it herself.

Chapter Six

CHANGES IN THE FAMILY

I had more things on my mind than Clara, my firstborn son Mike, was getting married. Mike was Clara's first grandchild, and we lived under the same roof. My feelings were conflicted, on one hand I wanted her there at my son's wedding, on the other hand, I wanted to enjoy the day and not have to worry about her being there and needing help. Clara was starting to be resistant to the idea of attending the wedding. I spoke with one of her daughter's who said, "Of course my mother is coming." I told her that I would be busy that day and she would have to take care of her mother at the wedding and reception. She agreed to that. By now Clara had made up her mind she was not going. Her argument was that the wedding was on a Friday, a dialysis day, and it was a two hour drive away. I told her that her dialysis could be switched to Saturday. Clara said she finds weddings boring and to sit that long in a car, then at the wedding and reception, then the return ride home was too much for her. Part of me had hurt feelings that she wasn't willing to put much effort forth to attend her grandson's wedding, feeling confident she would put that effort forth for one of her granddaughters. The other part of me was happy because I could enjoy my son's wedding without the distraction of my mother-in-law. Clara's other daughter said she would stay back to take care of her mother. I hated that I felt happier about that decision than sad, but it really did work out for the best.

We went down the day before the wedding for the rehearsal dinner, and then came home the morning after the wedding. I found when I would get a break from caring for Clara, the closer we would get to home, the tenser I would become. I had to mentally start preparing myself to go back into that role of caregiving. When we got home I was describing how everything went to Clara and she seemed to enjoy hearing about it. I excused myself to go unpack, and that is when the phone rang. "Michele, I had an accident." In my mind I was starting to call them an 'on purpose.' Reality slapped me in the face way too soon.

Mike wasn't leaving until Sunday morning for his honeymoon, and before leaving he called home to thank me and his Dad for all we did, and for the kind of parents we are. That made everything okay again. The joy of the wedding memories returned.

Soon thereafter, we got a call from Clara's assigned nurse from the Department of Aging. She was required to come out periodically to check on Clara's status, re-evaluate her need for care, etc. From an earlier visit she knew that my son was getting married and asked about that. I told her a bit about it, and then told her that it seems like every time we are away, the day after we return home Clara has an accident. I told her while it is annoying to deal with, it also makes me feel guilty that me going away has such a detrimental affect on her health. The nurse told me it was very likely Clara was doing it intentionally, as punishment. I could not believe that could be possible, that someone would actually soil themselves to make a point? The consistency of it happening, each time after we were away, made me start believing it was the case. That was information I wished I never knew. At least before when I would feel angry or frustrated, I would try to tell myself this also had to be difficult on Clara, not even having control over her own bodily functions. Now, even the possibility this was 'payback' for me getting a break away was hard information for me to swallow.

Time marches on and so does life. Winter was approaching, and Clara would always deteriorate some over the winter. She would typically get a cold that would last a good portion of the winter, and as a result become even weaker. The guys annual ski trip was fast approaching, and this would be the first trip all the guys were together since Mike was married. I started feeling a bit run down myself and before long I knew I had bronchitis. Unfortunately, it was December 31ˢᵗ when my temperature went up and all the doctor's offices had closed early. By the next day I was sicker than I ever remembered being with bronchitis before, and I had a strange looking rash on my arm. At first I thought the dog's claws had scratched my arm, but now I was noticing this scratch looked like tiny bumps. I felt so sick I stayed in our guest room, hoping Andy wouldn't catch what I had. My faithful companion Carly, would curl up and lay next to me, looking concerned when I had coughing spells that were hard to stop. She would only get up to go outside to the bathroom and then return right to bed with me. That's a loyal dog! Since it was January 1ˢᵗ, Andy was off work and took care of the house and his mother. The next day he had to go to work, and even though this was day three of running a 102+ degree temperature, Clara still required her care. Fortunately, it was not a dialysis day and I drove myself to the doctors. I was diagnosed with bronchitis and the flu. Then I slid up my shirt sleeve and said, "Oh yeah, I thought my dog scratched my arm, but now I'm noticing small bumps, what kind of rash is this?" Upon closer inspection the doctor said they were shingles. I left with a handful of prescriptions to get filled and could not wait to get back home to bed. I came home and got Clara her lunch, then crawled into bed, I felt rotten. I've been knocked down with sickness before, but Andy said this was the worst he had ever seen me. He wondered about leaving for their ski trip. I could not believe here was another ski trip and I was sick! Andy would pay for a nice condo for all the guys to stay in for this trip; it was his annual gift to them. So I would never even consider Andy staying home because others would be affected by that. The next day Clara would express concern about how terrible I sounded, but still expected the same amount of work from me for her care. When I was riding her to dialysis she commented on how terrible my cough sounded. Then she would ask me to run to her favorite soup place, another fifteen minutes away, to get her soup for after dialysis. I told her I would run to the local grocery store and get her soup and she turned her nose up to jarred soup. How did she get to this point in life where she couldn't see beyond herself, knowing how sick I was? Normally I would have ended up going and getting the soup

Conquers health issues.

Clara wanted, but grumbling to myself the entire way. This time, I physically just didn't have it; I needed to get back to bed. I told her it was the grocery store soup or nothing, and she agreed. My fever was back up, it was a damp, cold, rainy day and as I walked into the grocery store with chills from my fever, I thought of the weekend ahead with Clara. I got home, set the alarm for the time to leave to pick Clara up, and crawled into bed. The alarm rang much too quickly, I still had chills, but had to drag myself back out to pick up Clara. When I arrived Clara asked how I was feeling. I didn't even answer her at first because I thought if she really cared, she would not have been a snot about her soup. She asked again and I said, "Terrible." She said she figured that and was sorry I felt so bad. In the same breath she added she could not wait to get home to have her hot tea and soup. I asked Clara if her daughters knew that I had bronchitis, the flu and shingles and she said they did. That would baffle me that they would not volunteer to kick up their time with their mother. The next day my mother took Clara out for their usual lunch date, and that meant several hours in bed for me. When I woke up I went downstairs to find myself something to eat and make myself some hot tea. Carly started barking and when I looked out the front window I saw my mother coming down the driveway. She was driving like a maniac, flying down the driveway. When she got out of the car she had a grim look on her face, and I watched as she opened the door for Clara to help her inside. Clara looked like she was shook up. My first thought was, 'Clara pooped herself.' Then I thought, 'Michele, why do you always think that?' I went back to my boiling tea water but was wondering what was going on, something wasn't right. I wanted to investigate, but I knew once I stepped foot into Clara's apartment, she might start asking for something and I didn't want that. So I decided that I would keep an eye out for when my mother left. Normally when she would take Clara out to lunch, she would get her inside then leave, so I thought if she didn't leave in five minutes, then I would go over to investigate. Sure enough she didn't leave, and when I went over, Clara's front door and storm door were wide open despite the twenty degree temperature. There was no sign of Clara or my mother and I knew what that meant, they were in the bathroom. Instant anger welled up inside of me and I pulled out a pair of latex gloves and started walking towards the bathroom. At that my mother emerged and with authority said, "Michele, get back to bed." I said, "Clara pooped herself didn't she?" My mother again ordered me back to my house in bed. I said it wasn't her responsibility to clean Clara up and went to close her front door. My mother said she could not handle the smell, and re-opened the front door. She also knew she could not clean up Clara; she was starting with the dry heaves from the smell in the car. Clara had the accident on the car ride home and my Mom had to put the windows down despite the cold temperature because of the odor. My mother called my sister-in-law Maria and Maria met them at Clara's apartment and she was cleaning Clara up. My mother was getting out fresh clothes for Clara to put on. I said it wasn't their responsibility and insisted that I would finish it up. Maria must have heard me talking, came out and assured me she had everything under control and would not permit me to take one step closer and for me to get back to bed. I listened but felt sad and furious at the same time. It was bad enough this was my life, but Clara was my mother-in-law, now my sister-in-law and mother are involved with this vile mess. Where are Clara's daughters? Why was no one stepping up? Why is it my family stepping up? The heat coming from my body was not just from my fever at this point. I was absolutely beside myself that Clara messed her pants in my mother's brand new car. Where that may sound uncompassionate on my part, it was because Clara ate creamed soup, which always causes her stomach upset and diarrhea. Knowing the affect that creamed soups had on her, I felt it was the height of selfishness for her to continue to consume it, since she was not the one that had to clean up the mess. After my mother and Maria took care of Clara, Maria cleaned up the mess it made in my mother's car.

I could not wait to tell Andy what his mother did. It's funny how that was always important for me to do. Since I felt Clara did not want to inconvenience her daughters by asking them to help with her care while I was recovering, I told Clara with her compromised immune system with being on dialysis, it was not in her best interest to have close contact with me. Once I expressed to Clara that she could become gravely ill by having close contact with me and that she would have to ask her daughters to help over the next week, she said she would have them look after her. Although I was truthful in what I was saying, I thought it was sad that it was only when Clara felt her health was in danger that she would ask them for the extra help. By now the small bumps on my arm had grown into a disgusting scabby mess about an inch wide and eight inches long. It was cracked and oozing and I could not imagine my arm ever recovering without a significant scar. I was on so many prescriptions; an anti-viral medicine, an anti-biotic, a decongestant, an expectorant, an inhaler and ibuprofen. It seemed like the shingles kept breaking out in new places each day. I returned to the doctor to find out I had an allergic reaction to one of the medications, but which one? Trying to figure that out delayed my recovery, I was sick for a month. I only had that extra help for one week, and at least after that, while I wasn't recovered, I had improved. I had a talk with Clara about the selfishness of her eating creamed soups knowing the affect it had on her. Months later, to my great surprise, the scar from the shingles actually faded away completely.

While this winter was hard on me, it was not problem free for Clara either. Clara always had a hard time making it through the winter without a lingering head cold. We both were happy when the warm spring weather appeared. Clara was approaching five years on dialysis and many would comment on how remarkable it was that Clara was still alive. I would give my running joke that I was told Clara would only live for two years on dialysis, and here it was almost five, I should have gotten that in writing. Yes, I know it is <u>sick humor</u>, but <u>whatever it took to keep going</u>!

By this time Mike was married and out of state, Zack involved with college, so Andy and I had more opportunities for travel. We had our annual April trip to New York for a long weekend to celebrate our wedding anniversary. Andy won another five day trip from his job, this time to Arizona the beginning of May. Mike and Tanya wanted us all to go to the Bahamas for a long weekend the end of May. Then in August we had our annual beach trip with my family. I could not believe all the traveling we had lined up. Then friends of ours were organizing a group to go on a Caribbean cruise in December. I felt greedy having so many trips planned but thought it was cool that we were at a point in our lives where we could travel; well except for Clara and Carly. For the New York and Arizona trips Zack could arrange his college schedule to still care for the dog. Clara wanted to stay in her apartment, so it was a matter of having her cared for during the day and Zack would put her to bed in the evening. Her daughters helped a bit more with that. Of course, even away we would have to call Zack each night close to Clara's bed time on his cell phone to remind him to put his grandmother to bed. We kept the December cruise quiet until after our August beach trip. We thought of the problems we had the past two years with vacation time and knew the increased amount of travel would not be greeted happily. With the cruise being the second week of December, I felt confident with us traveling during a busy holiday month; it would be met with even more resistance.

Come September I broke the news to Clara about the cruise. Then I came up with the idea of having Clara arrange for her own care. Rather than me getting the phone call at the last minute for the arrangements I made, I thought let Clara take care of making arrangements with her own daughters. I had a hard time not getting involved. Clara mentioned to me she told her one daughter about the cruise. She related her reply was that is a busy time for her and she wouldn't be available for anything extra. I would remind Clara to be sure to make her own arrangements. We were taking my mother along on the cruise as a thank you for all the luncheons she arranged each week for Clara, so Clara knew she wasn't available to help care for her. Andy would ask me about the arrangements and I told him it was up to his mother and the more I asked, the more it involved me. He said his worry was we would have a problem days before the cruise and he didn't want that stress before leaving on our first cruise. About three weeks before the cruise, I started pressing Clara regarding what her arrangements were. She was trying to involve anyone but her own daughters. When I asked her why, she said they were not available. I was not sure if it was their words or Clara not wanting to ask them. That would puzzle me how it could be so easy for her to ask her daughter-in-law to wipe her butt but not ask her own daughter for help in her care. Zack was going to be home the week of the cruise, but he said he would be cramming; studying for finals. He said he could care for the dog, but didn't want the responsibility of caring for his grandmother this time. Since he tends to study late into the night, he said he didn't want to be in the middle of studying, to have to stop to put his grandmother to bed. On one hand that seemed ridiculous, but on the other hand I thought we should be able to go away for a week and not have to be the only family members involved with Clara's care. Zack was not a stranger to helping with Clara. The times when Clara would not be able to get up by herself and Zack was home, he would stop what he was doing to assist. Once when Andy met us at the car to help his mother in the house after dialysis, she demanded Zack help her. Andy is quite strong and was more than capable. Once Clara made up her mind there was no changing it. To me it was actually quite funny. Neither Andy nor Zack found the humor in it. Zack was in the middle of completing an assignment for college, and while he was accommodating to his grandmother, it was enough to break his concentration. I decided not to argue with him about his decision.

The week before the cruise, I asked Clara if she had made her final care arrangements. She told me what they were, which involved very little of her own daughters. Then she said, "Since Zack will be home, he can put me to bed at night." I said, "No, he can't." That rattled Clara. I told her that Zack had finals to study for and that we should be able to go away for a week and between her two daughters, they should be able to do what we do the rest of the year. I pointed out even though we had traveled a lot that past year, when you consider the amount of days in a year, and that we had been gone less than twenty days so far, it wasn't too much to ask. I was determined to stick to my guns on this one; I guess I felt like I had a point to prove. Then Clara looked dejected and I felt bad. I told her I was sorry that the cruise was bad timing and that I didn't want her to feel like she was a burden to us. I expressed that I felt it was reasonable for her to ask her own daughters to help out; after all, she is their mother. Clara said she understood and that we deserved to go on the cruise and I didn't need to apologize for it. When she would say stuff like that it would make me feel like crap for being hard nosed. I went back to my side of the house, and later came over with a cup of hot tea as a peace offering. I heard Clara on the phone with one of her daughter's saying, "She said Zack can't put me to bed, I guess I'll sleep in my chair." I tipped toed back to my side and felt so torn. I thought I would let Zack know the outcome and see if he would reconsider. Was this a principle really worth fighting for? Why did she always want it easiest on her own daughters? I waited a few minutes then went back with a cheerful, "I have some hot tea for you" and Clara was off the phone. She told me that her daughter that lives a mile from our house would come over each night to put her to bed. That was a relief to me and Clara.

Before we knew it, it was time to fly to Puerto Rico for our cruise. I retyped all of Clara's medical information to update it, made up another chart of Clara's medicines, and filled her daily pill dispensers. We were going to be gone nine days, so at first I thought I would buy some extra pill dispensers. Then I thought this was a good opportunity for Clara's daughter to become familiar with her mother's medicines, and with the detailed list it would be easy to refill her weekly dispenser. We were off on the cruise and had a great time. Unfortunately, toward the end of the cruise I got sick. I woke up the last full day of the cruise with a tickle in my throat, and by evening I was running a fever and was coughing like I had bronchitis. Andy and I were both amazed at how sick I became so quickly. That night we packed our bags and put them outside our cabin door as instructed and I crawled into bed. During the night I woke up with chills and a horrible headache, and although I didn't have a thermometer, I'm confident my temperature was well over 103. I knew if I took ibuprofen, it would help some, but I can't take it on an empty stomach, and I didn't have the energy to get some food. Andy was sleeping soundly and I didn't want to disturb him. As I laid there miserable, I thought when I got home that there was no way I was going to get any more help with Clara. I wanted to be home in my own bed but the thought of going home to my routine was dreadful. Morning came, and I got myself together to vacate our cabin by the mandatory 8:00 a.m. time. I felt horrible, but reminded myself that it could be worse. I thought of the year before when I had shingles, the flu and bronchitis all at one time. I did eat some dry toast for breakfast, took some ibuprofen, and within an hour started to get a little relief from my symptoms. We were able to pay to have our plane tickets switched to an earlier time. We arrived home to frigid temperatures and an icy snow. Not thinking, I had packed all of my shoes and had sandals on and a sweater. Fortunately, my brother picked us up and cranked the heat up for us. I got home and greeted Carly, who was delirious with excitement that we finally came home. It was late, and Clara was already put to bed. The next morning, I went over, and none of Clara's pill dispensers were filled. To me it looked like just enough were filled until I got home. Being sick, I had no patience for that and exaggerated the reason why in my mind. I felt like it was deliberately done to make a point that nothing more than the bare minimum was going to be done. There was debris lying around and I told Clara that I got the point loud and clear from her daughter that she was not happy about our trip. I had a major attitude. Clara asked what I was talking about and I was all too eager to tell her about none of the pill dispensers being filled, although I was courteous enough to fill them up before I left. There were empty grocery bags and tags that were pulled off of clothes on the floor. Who was going to take care of these things? Clara wasn't able. I was spitting mad. Part of it was the frustration of coming home sick and having to go right back into the caregiver's role. Another part was the ongoing resentment I felt toward Clara's daughters. I left for the doctor's and sure enough had bronchitis again. I came home and crawled into bed. I was having a bad coughing spell when the phone rang and I thought there was no sense in answering it, because I couldn't stop coughing. Whoever called left a message. When my coughing calmed down and I checked my voice mail, I had a nasty message from Clara's daughter to call her at work. Clara must have called her daughter to either report my complaint or to scold her for leaving things the way she did. I called her back, and she was furious at my assumption that she purposely did not fill her mother's medicine dispenser. She pointed out I had returned from my trip hours earlier than I had originally said and she had planned to refill them that day. I apologized if I came to a wrong conclusion and then she proceeded to angrily tell me how she has to get up for work at 5:00 a.m. and it was quite a burden for her to have to come out at night to come over to put her mother to bed. I commented that is what we have to do all the time; we have to revolve our lives around her mother's bedtime. Then she got really hyper and said, "Yeah, but you didn't have to come out at eleven at night in the cold nighttime air, then go home wide awake and have a hard time falling back to sleep." At this point I asked her if her mother had told her I had come home sick and she said she mentioned it. I said, "You know that I'm sick but you still called to yell at me?" She said she wasn't yelling, but didn't appreciate being accused of not filling the pill dispenser on purpose. She added she hated how I always act like I do everything. I was surprised that she said that. I retorted that I hate how every time that she or her sister do something for their own mother, they act as if they are doing me a big favor. With that we ended the call and I went back to bed, coughing and hacking away. Somehow, the thought of her being inconvenienced made me happy, like it was her just due. At first I was feeling sorry for myself for having to deal with this crap, and then felt happy that Clara's daughter felt like she had to deal with my crap! Then it was time to get back up to care for Clara, so I guess I didn't have the last laugh after all. The delightful cruise was over and it was back to reality.

I bounced back rather quickly from my bronchitis, but Clara wasn't doing well at all. She was becoming weaker, asking for more and more help in getting out of her chair. I would remind her that due to my injuries, I really needed her to get up herself because it was too hard on me. She would try again and sometimes she could get up, but other times she really could not. Despite me swearing I would not hurt my body one more time by picking her up, I would pick her up. There was no choice, she physically was unable. Sometimes, Zack would be home and I would call on him to help. He is so strong he could pick her up like a rag doll. I was always grateful for the times he was home when Clara needed help.

--

Chapter Seven

THE GRADUAL DECLINE

As we went into the month of January, Clara seemed to get her winter head cold a bit early. Something about Clara just didn't seem right to me and I was worrying about what was going on. I expressed my concern to Clara's other daughter, not the one I had the spat with weeks before. In the past when Clara would start with congestive heart failure, this daughter could actually hear it in her mother's voice when she would talk over the telephone before I would hear it. She said she was coming down the next day for her weekly visit and would observe her. She agreed she seemed a bit weaker but didn't think she had the chest congestion yet. By the weekend Clara seemed worse to me, having more and more difficulty getting up. She had several bouts of diarrhea, not once making it to the bathroom because she was too weak to get up out of her lazy girl chair. While I wasn't thrilled with having to clean her up throughout the day, my concern for Clara was growing. Carly, our dog delighted in all of these accidents. When she would follow me over to Clara's apartment, she would sniff Clara's butt, in true dog fashion as I escorted her to the bathroom. Clara and I would be yelling at Carly to stop. Once I got Clara in the bathroom, I would have to get Carly back to our side of the house and shut the door. Even with Clara wearing an adult diaper, it was still a mess to clean up. We would keep small trash bags under her bathroom sink so we could wrap the soiled items up tightly. There were a number of times that Carly got into the trash and got out the small bag with the soiled adult diaper in it. I would find a chewed up messy diaper in my front yard!! I always loved having to clean Clara's poop up twice!

As a result of my ongoing concern for Clara, I called the other daughter, the one I had the spat with. I left her a message asking her to call me after her visit with her mother on Saturday. I wanted to know what she thought after observing her Mom. She did not call me, which I of course read into. On Monday I called her at work to see her feelings on her mother's condition. She said she didn't think her mother was doing that bad. She thought it was just her usual winter deterioration. I was still convinced that something was wrong. Another week had gone by and Clara now had this hacking cough that sounded deep in her chest. She was extremely weak now. It reminded me of six years before when she had pneumonia and was too weak to hold up her head. It was time to leave for dialysis and Clara could not get up from her chair at all. I helped lift her up wondering how we would ever make it to the car. As we walked to the car she was very unstable on her feet and I think we both quietly feared she would fall. After just a few steps, we would have to stop for Clara to catch her breath. It was an ordeal getting Clara in the car and once we did I told Clara that I was concerned for her and I felt she was worried too. At first Clara just listened. I told her that I had not seen that much weakness in her since her bout with pneumonia and my concern was that after her dialysis treatment she would be in an even weaker condition. I continued that I know how much she hates the hospital, but that I hate to see her suffer if something in her body is out of balance that we can fix and give her relief. I told her I thought it would be best that after dialysis, we would plan on going to the emergency room to help figure out why she was so weak. When Clara agreed to my plan I knew how scared she was. I told her I would call her doctor and let him know what our plans were. It was quite a chore getting Clara out of the car into dialysis and into her treatment chair but she seemed emotionally and mentally prepared for going to the hospital. With Clara, that was more than half of the battle. I finally got in touch with her doctor and expressed my concerns. He was at another dialysis center that day. I told him I was quite concerned that something was seriously wrong with Clara. I even commented if she had something like cancer, I would never want her to be burdened with that knowledge. I was a bit cautious about the possibility of opening a can of worms like that. However, I knew in my heart there was something going on with Clara that could not be ignored. The doctor said he didn't think she had cancer. I asked him if he thought she was dying and to my surprise and disappointment he laughed at my question and then said no. I reminded him that she had been on dialysis for over five and a half years now, asking if her body could be breaking down. He said no. I again emphasized I was certain something was seriously wrong. He replied that her last labs didn't show anything significant. I commented that blood work doesn't show everything and she has agreed to go to the hospital and that we needed to figure out if she had something treatable. Up to this conversation, I felt like I had a very good working relationship with Clara's doctor. I was shocked when he said that the emergency room isn't a place to dump my mother-in-law off and Medicare would not pay for endless unnecessary tests. I was offended at the suggestion this was not about my concern for my mother-in-law. I firmly assured him this was not a case of me trying to get my mother-in-law off my hands to give me a break. That I am involved in her daily care, and I'm saying something is very, very wrong with her. She was extremely weak, she had hardly any appetite, what she did eat caused diarrhea and she is too weak to get up and get to the bathroom. The doctor still seemed unconcerned, and a bit apathetic. This conversation took place on Monday, and he said he would be at her dialysis center on Wednesday, and he would talk with her and check on her then. I could not believe it, I left Clara at dialysis convinced going to the hospital was in her best interest, and I knew once I picked her up and took her home, that opportunity for her to agree to go to the hospital would be gone. On Wednesday, Clara's daughter came down as normal, and now she was concerned with the chest congestion her mother had. Later that evening when Clara got home from dialysis I asked her if the doctor examined her. She said he had written down a suggestion. When I picked up his note it said, "Give Clara a can of Glucerna protein drink each morning." I looked at Clara and asked, "Did you tell him I have been giving you a can of Glucerna in the morning for the past year?" Clara went into her playing dumb routine and said, "Oh, do you?" She then continued that the more she thought about it, she really didn't think she was sick but she was depressed because of the days being shorter. She added that her winter cold came earlier than normal and come spring time, things would be better. I knew my golden opportunity to find out what was wrong with Clara had past and I would not get her to agree again to go to the hospital. At this point, going to the hospital was out of the question since her doctor felt it was unnecessary. By Friday, it was ridiculous trying to get Clara to the car for dialysis. It was as if the bottoms of her feet were rounded from carrying so much fluid and she could barely balance herself. It took about fifteen minutes to get her to the car. Once home from dialysis, it was even worse. That evening she called her daughter and said she would not be going out on Saturday, she wasn't feeling well. Saturday continued with her daily diarrhea and weakness. I didn't know what it was, but in my heart I knew something was very, very wrong. I felt absolutely helpless and angry with Clara's doctor when I even thought of his suggestion that I was trying to dump Clara off for a break. Sure there were times I felt like I needed a break, but never would I try to have her admitted unnecessarily. For the quality of care he knew I provided Clara, which he had often commented on himself, it was extremely insulting and I was mad. Sunday morning Clara just looked pathetic. In the morning she had no appetite. She drank her protein drink for the nutritive value, and before long that went right through her. We had switched from her having coffee to hot tea to see if that would help stop the diarrhea. By mid afternoon Clara called that she had another accident. Honestly, I could not imagine how anything was even left in her system to cause diarrhea. I went over and Clara was just a lump in her chair. I talked to her tenderly and told her that I was very concerned about her and she softly said, "I know." It was obvious she was scared and that she knew something was wrong and could not ignore it any longer. I told her that we have waited as long as we could wait, but she needed to go to the hospital. She immediately agreed. I told her that after I washed her up, I was going to dress her, and then I was going to take her to the hospital. She could not continue on as weak as she was. Clara said she was ready to go to the hospital after I washed her up. She was so weak; I had to stand behind Clara with my stomach pressed to her back as I wrapped my arms around her waist from behind. With her having a mess in her pants, it wasn't ideal, but she truly needed the help. We slowly walked in unison to the bathroom and she said she wanted to sit on the toilet for a few minutes to see if she was emptied out. Once seated, I told her I would be back in a few minutes. I marched back to my side of the house and Andy asked if she had another accident and when I said yes, he said he was going to call his sister, it was time for her to come over since she felt like everything was okay. I told him not to do that, I would clean her up, but that I would no longer take 'no' for an answer, she was going to the hospital. I then got on the phone and called Clara's daughter that lives about a half hour away and told her what I was doing. She was fully supportive and said she would meet us at the emergency room. I went back to Clara, and she was ready to get in the shower. She was so weak it was a challenge for her to lift her foot the two and a half inches to clear the shower ledge even with my help. She held onto the handicap hand rails as I undressed her in the shower. Once I rinsed the feces away, I had to get into the shower with her to help hold her up. She then had to sit down on the shower seat as she was too weak to continue standing. I'm in the shower thinking how I cannot believe the doctor had let things go this far. Once she sat down, she had a bit more diarrhea, so when she was able, I helped her back up so I could re-wash the area. I draped a towel over her chest to prevent a chill until we could get to her bed for her to sit on the side so I could dress her. She said she was not able to lift her foot up to get out of the shower. I'm thinking, 'Crap, what do I do now?' Andy and Zack were home, but Clara would be humiliated for them to have them help her out of the shower. Plus I could not even leave her to ask them for help. I told her that I could not get her out of the shower by myself and she could not get out of the shower by herself, but together we could do it. I pressed my stomach back again into her back, put my hands around her waist and slid my left foot under her left foot and helped lift it out as she hung onto the hand rail. With me standing right up against Clara's back, I could not see my feet or her feet so it was a bit tricky, but her left foot was out. I said, "We make a good team." Clara said, "I can't get my other foot out." I said, "Remember, we are a team, we can do it together." I was trying to put my foot under her right foot as she was trying to lift her foot out over the shower stall lip. Then she said,

"I'm going to fall." With absolutely desperation in my voice I said, "NO YOU ARE NOT, DON'T FALL." In the past when Clara would think she was going to fall, she would allow herself to fall on purpose, so she could somewhat control her fall. I had been in the situation before when this happened when I was trying to hold Clara up and she just becomes dead weight. When Clara uttered, "I'm going to fall" I knew if I did not convince her she was not going to fall, she would become dead weight. Clara repeated those words a second time and I said now with panic, "No you're not, no, you're not" and as I could feel her releasing her body I was desperately trying to hold her up and she was slowly falling. It all happened quickly yet it seemed in slow motion. As Clara's right foot stayed hooked on the shower stall lip, I was desperately trying to let it out with my foot. Clara went down and I heard a popping noise. Although it was a noise I had never heard before, I knew immediately it was the sound of a bone that snapped in two. I'm still trying to hold her body weight up, and her right leg is caught under her body and is now in an unnatural position. Clara said, "I think I broke my leg." I calmly said that she did, as my fight was now over with holding her vertical, I gently stroked her cheek and said, "Don't worry, it will be okay, I'll take care of you." Then I turned my head to where I thought my voice would project the best and screamed, "Andy, get over here." Then I would gently stroke Clara's face some more and try to reassure her, then scream for Andy to hurry up. She probably thought I was an absolute nut switching from calm and reassuring to hysterically yelling! The very thing I was trying to avoid happened anyway. I re-draped the towel to cover Clara as much as I could and I asked Andy to help me lift her to get her leg out from under her. He said he didn't think we should move her, you are never supposed to move an injured person. Normally I would have agreed, but at this point I knew she had a broken bone, moving her would not change that. I did not want to further complicate things by her leg having no circulation with all her body weight on it, and I felt we had no choice. With authority I said we had to get the pressure off of her leg and Andy agreed. It was obvious the femur, or thigh bone that was broken. I stayed behind Clara holding her up so she didn't fall backwards and hit her head too. After Andy helped get her leg out, I said to call 911. He did and was placed on hold. It was probably for a minute or two,

broke her leg !

but seemed forever. When he finished I told him he had to come back in the bathroom and hold his mother up, I physically couldn't hold her up anymore. Andy stood behind his mother holding her up, keeping his eyes closed so he wouldn't see his mother partially naked. I had flashbacks to when Clara had the stroke when I thought that was it, her life as we knew it was over, but I was wrong. I knew this time there was no such room for error. Clara would have to go to a nursing home at least for rehabilitation of her broken leg, and we still did not know what was wrong with her that lead to this fall. It was all so very sad. Andy wisely asked me to get a blanket to lie over his mother, I hadn't even thought of that. Then I noticed when she fell she had a bit more diarrhea. I thought all of this was for nothing! I was cleaning her up so she could go to the hospital, and she was going to end up going to the hospital soiled anyway, now with a broken leg. I was wet and soiled and told Andy that I was going to hurry up and change my clothes before the paramedics arrived and let Zack know what was going on. As I hurried out of the bathroom Clara's phone rang. Thinking it may be 911 calling back I answered it. It was Clara's daughter that lives nearby. She said, "What's going on, I got a call you are taking Mom to the hospital." I told her she fell and broke her leg and she responded anxiously, "Please don't tell me that." I'm thinking, 'what do you mean don't tell me that?' It was what happened, I told her I had to hang up and change my wet clothes before the paramedics arrived. We live off of a dirt and gravel road and it had been snowing and we could see the paramedics and ambulance drive past the turn off to our driveway. Zack ran down our long driveway to wave them back, and the ambulance got stuck in the snow. The paramedics made it down rather quickly and started assessing Clara right away. Another one asked for her current medications and conditions, and I was glad I had her updated medical information in that vial in the refrigerator. Her daughter came in and asked what happened. When I explained it she said, "Why didn't you call me? I would have come over and helped you." I knew she was upset about her mother, so I didn't reply what I was thinking. I couldn't believe that she believed that she would really do that. I also felt like calling Clara's doctor and saying, 'See, I told you something was wrong and you didn't listen, and now look what happened.' I still had so much anger towards Clara's doctor for not taking my concerns seriously. I was so glad that Andy had earlier shoveled a clear path to Clara's door and down our sidewalk. As a result Clara could more easily be carried out by gurney. I was able to dress her from the waist up, but we wrapped her bottom half up in a blanket. I felt horrible for Clara and as she was wheeled out, I knew the chances of her ever returning through that door were slim. We drove over to the hospital and it was an absolute zoo. Clara was sitting in the ambulance bay waiting for a place to be put; everything was full on this snowy Sunday afternoon. We were not allowed back to see her and were limited to the waiting area. Clara is not good about speaking up for herself and I mentioned that to someone because I wanted Clara to have something for pain. In time the nurse said that only one person could go back. I yielded to her children although I really wanted to be by her side. One daughter went back, and then another was able to go back. It wasn't long before they needed me to provide information on Clara's medications so I got to see her. She was in and out of it. It was heartbreaking for me to witness. I went outside of the cubicle and told Clara's assigned nurse that while she was brought in by ambulance for a broken bone, we were planning on coming to the hospital before that. I pleaded with her to ask at least for a chest x-ray and explained her chest congestion has increased significantly over the past few days. The nurse seemed to listen when I said that even before the break, something was very wrong with Clara. I went back to the waiting room, and Andy went back with his sisters. This went off and on until an orthopedic came in and asked some questions about her medical history none of them knew. Andy came to the waiting room and waved me back, and he introduced me to the doctor as his wife, and his mother's caregiver. In my view, it looked like her daughters flashed a look of objection to that title. I tried to be considerate of what they were going through, but I thought I'm not going to correct Andy because there was nothing to correct. I asked him if they did a chest x-ray and he said they did and there was quite a bit of fluid around her heart. Later he told me privately there was an unknown mass in her left lung that would have to be looked into once she was stabilized. X-rays revealed Clara broke her femur in half, that news was not a surprise to me. However, I did not realize that the femur is the biggest bone in your body. In order for Clara to heal, surgery would be needed. A rod would be placed in her leg and attached to each side of the broken bone with screws. The problem was she was not stable enough for surgery. She was on Coumadin, a blood thinner and her blood was too thin for surgery, in addition to the chest congestion. She would need a couple of days and would be kept as comfortable as possible with pain medication. At that point they were waiting for a bed to open up on the floor for Clara to be admitted. Andy told his sisters they could leave; we would stay with her until she was put in her room. One left, the other one stayed even though she had to get up 5:00 am for work the next day, she just wasn't ready to leave her mother yet. When Clara was transported to her room, she left, and Andy and I followed her up. Clara was still in and out of it, and as she got to the floor, the nurse was asking us some questions. It was now quite late, and we told Clara we were leaving and would be back the next morning. Clara said, "I'm sorry I caused such problems." I had to hold back the tears as we assured her that we were sorry for what happened and what she was going through, she had no reason to apologize.

On the way home I thought about all the times she would leave her used tissues in her chair. From time to time, I would ask her if she could please put them in the wastebasket right next to her chair, but I would always find her used, rolled up tissues in the sides of her chair. Those were the little irritations of day to day life that she never seemed bothered by, and here on something so tragic, that was out of her control she is saying she is sorry. When we got home that night I asked Andy if he was okay. He said he felt sad for his mother, but was okay. I told him I was going to stay up for a while and would come to bed later. After he went to sleep, I went in the guest room, buried my head in a pillow and bawled my eyes out. I felt so bad that Clara fell on my watch. I felt angry that I didn't listen to my instincts and demand Clara be evaluated before this traumatic injury. My anger towards Clara's doctor for having such a cavalier attitude and even chuckling at my concern was becoming overwhelming. I knew Clara's life as we knew it was over. That night I mourned the end of Clara, even though she was still alive.

The doctor confirmed my earlier suspicion that after surgery, she would be discharged from the hospital to a nursing home for rehabilitation. It would be eight to twelve weeks before she could come home. In my mind and heart,

I knew Clara would not do well in a nursing home setting, even though I was already mentally planning on visiting her daily. Then there was the matter of what was wrong with Clara to cause this weakness in the first place. What was the unknown mass in her lung? I imagined Clara in a nursing home dying a slow, painful death. I prayed if she was going to die, if it was reasonable to ask, to help her die quickly. I felt all of my hard work in Clara's behalf went down the drain, as if it was all for nothing. I wondered if her daughters were mad at me for Clara falling when I was caring for her. I wondered how Andy felt about it. It was a long hard night, but I kept all of these feelings to myself and would plant a smile on my face for everyone else. The next morning, after Andy left for work, I decided to work on a funeral program for Clara. My thinking was, if she dies it would be hard to write a nice obituary for her. I wanted an obituary that when read, people would learn something about Clara they did not know before. I knew even if it was not immediately needed, it would be needed in the months ahead. I thought if I waited, I would be so drained emotionally I would not be able to do it justice. I actually called a long time friend of Clara's, that I am a friend with now, to ask her if my recollection of what Clara had previous related to me was accurate. Other than that phone call, I did not dare tell anyone what I had been working on. I'm a planner, so for me it made sense but I knew for her family it would be offensive. When I arrived at the hospital, I was happy to see that the pain medication really knocked Clara out, as long as she was sleeping, she wasn't suffering. By Tuesday, two days later Clara was still not stable enough for surgery. Even though she was off the Coumadin, her blood continued to thin without explanation. Also, Clara had internal bleeding from the break. Her condition was worsening. I had been to the hospital for a visit and once I got home the doctor called wanting my approval for a particular treatment that she felt was necessary for Clara. It was not a treatment I was comfortable with and I asked some questions. The house doctor got a bit nasty with me and insinuated that I was jeopardizing Clara's life. I told her that I could not give permission to a treatment I did not feel was in Clara's best interest. I asked if there were any alternative treatment options. This doctor demanded my approval and would not discuss any treatment options. I refused approval until I knew all of Clara's treatment options.

The doctor asked if there was another family member she could talk with. I told her Clara's daughter would be there in two hours and she could discuss it with her if she preferred and see if she would grant permission if she deemed it necessary. With that the phone call ended. This doctor apparently went to Clara's room and convinced her this treatment was of life or death urgency and Clara gave her verbal approval. Since she was on the pain medication, they needed another family member to agree to it. Now a nurse called to speak with me, said she was at the bedside with Clara and the doctor when Clara agreed to the treatment. At that point, I felt like I had the right to fight for Clara, but I was not going to fight Clara. If I was right or wrong in my opinion was not the issue now, it was supporting what Clara wanted. She had the right to make her own choice. I called Andy at work and told him what his mother wanted. He was surprised at how stressed I was by giving permission for this treatment in his mother's behalf since it was really her decision and not mine. Clara actually had a durable health care power of attorney and Andy was listed as her health care agent. He decided after our phone call, that he was going to invoke his authority as her health care agent and start making his mother's medical decisions; I was out of the equation. Finally, it was such a relief!

That evening Andy was going to the hospital to see his mother after work and I knew at least his one sister would be there. I went over to a friend's house for one hour and did not even take my cell phone. I wanted a break from life; I did not want to be contacted. Afterward, I went over to my mother's. Since we live next door to one another, Zack saw me drive over there before coming home. He came over and said, "Call Dad on his cell phone immediately." I called and asked, "What is going on?" Andy replied, "Mom coded." That was all he said. I hopped in my car and hurried over to the hospital. I tried to brace myself for anything. I analyzed his words, "Mom coded." I thought if she was not revived he probably would have said, 'Mom died.' So I reasoned that she must have been resuscitated. I wasn't sure so I tried to prepare myself to be a support system. Andy and his sister were in the hallway and there were a team of doctor's surrounding Clara's bed. She was alive. Andy filled me in on what happened. He had asked his Mom if she wanted him to throw the tissue away in her hand and she said, "No thanks." Moments later he noticed she was not breathing and called for help. She was resuscitated. It was a terrible thing for Andy and his sister to witness. I went over to Clara and stood next to her. I was mad because I felt like Clara was bullied into this treatment that her hospital doctor insisted on, and Clara obviously had a reaction to it. The hospital's critical care doctor said that a toxic level of narcotics built up in Clara's system. Since her kidneys are non-functioning, and she was getting narcotic pain medication every four hours that it was like a drug overdose. I wasn't buying it. That would have been more plausible if there wasn't a special team in her room, filling out paperwork indicating there was a reaction to the treatment the doctor had done just a couple of hours before Clara coded. Andy said later he could not believe that his mother was on monitors, yet the hospital staff failed to notice she coded until he called out for help. He wondered if he wasn't there; if the hospital would have noticed in time to save her life. I said, "I wonder if you really did her a favor." I should have just thought that, but stupidly said it out loud. I could see my words hurt him. I did not mean that in a hurtful way, but I remained convinced that Clara had a terrible future ahead of her, ending in death. I thought of my prayer about Clara dying quickly and I wondered if Andy screwed that up. I kept my mouth shut about it after that, and just thought things. After that, the doctor would only give Clara over the counter Tylenol for her pain. The poor thing was in agony. The next night my son Mike drove up from Virginia to visit his grandmother and got to see some of his cousins who were visiting at the same time. Clara seemed thrilled to have her grandchildren around, even with the pain she was dealing with. The doctor that followed Clara's care during dialysis was a nephrologist (kidney specialist), but Clara also needed a general practitioner to monitor all of her care as an inpatient. I gave the nurse the name of the original doctor that saw Clara after the eye doctor, way back when, that met us in his office on a Sunday morning for the first time to see Clara. He had managed Clara's care up to dialysis. The hospital contacted him. When he walked into Clara's hospital room he said, "Michele, how are you?!" He gave me a hug. I was shocked that he remembered my name. Andy and both of his sisters were in the room. He told them that he was always impressed with the care that I gave Clara and that he seldom sees a daughter care for her own mother the way I took care of my mother-in-law. As kind as his words were, I was not sure how Clara's daughters would take them. To my happy surprise, it seemed like the first time they saw me in a good light. After a while, one even got up and offered her seat to me since I was standing. When we left after our visit, I told Andy I think I like it better when his sisters view me as a pain in the butt and suspiciously. Their kindness threw me off and felt confusing. By Thursday, it was four days since her break and she still was not as stable as was hoped. The orthopedic said the surgery just could not wait. At this point, the risks of waiting another day outweighed the risks of surgery. Besides, Clara could not continue to lay there suffering. Surgery was scheduled late in the day, around 5:30 p.m. Andy and I, and both of her daughters were all there well before the surgery. Clara was always nervous before any procedure, but she didn't seem especially nervous before this major operation. We all followed her gurney as she was wheeled down to the operating area. As the nurses wheeled her into the first part of the operating entrance, we were told we could continue with her. We stood in this hallway a few minutes until the anesthesiologist appeared. He had lots of questions, but seemed like a kind, older man. As he explained in detail to Clara what his role was, including how he would put a breathing tube down her throat, I stood there thinking that he should shut up. In the past Clara always deferred things to me at doctor's appointments because she didn't like to hear the details. I thought I should tell him that was too much information, but then reasoned that three of her children are standing there and saying nothing, Clara seemed okay with it, and I'm sure it was his responsibility to inform her. I wanted to protect her from hearing it but couldn't. Within minutes, we were told to say our goodbyes and go to the waiting area, that someone would see us after her surgery and let us know when we could visit with her in recovery.

We all walked to the waiting area, and some time later I excused myself to go to the cafeteria to get a cold drink. Andy said he would stay; he had brought stuff from work that had to be done. Both of Clara's daughters stood up and said they would walk down with me. We walked to the cafeteria like a family; I think it was the first time I could ever remember it feeling like that. Normally it seemed like us and them, always a division. I thought of all the times following Clara's various doctors' appointments I would always call each of them to let them know what had happened, and it never seemed to really connect us.

For the first time, I felt like we were connected and I was actually accepted. It was almost strange to me how good that felt. I had always thought I put most effort forth for Andy's benefit; he had been more like a father to his sisters when they were growing up, than a brother. Since their father abandoned the family when Andy was eight years old, and he was the oldest child, a lot of responsibility fell on him. As we married and his sisters got older, at first he felt hurt at the lack of interest they seemed to have in their relationship with him. I would remind him that is typical; as young ones grow up they get involved in their own interests. I felt since we were older than them, it was more of our responsibility to reach out and stay in touch. Now, we are walking to the hospital cafeteria and I am delighted to feel connected. I wondered why that was so important to me. As we walked we laughed and it was probably the best experience I had ever had with the two of them. We came back to the waiting room for a rather extended wait. Most of the other people that were in the waiting room when we first arrived had already received news of their loved ones and had cleared out.

Soon my brother Jim and Maria walked in. We could hardly believe it since they were leaving in the morning for a weekend trip. It broke up the boredom. Then my other brother and his wife, Tom and Barb came in. They were going away on the same trip with Jim and Maria, so we never expected them to show up at the hospital around 8:00 p.m. at night. Moments later, close friends of ours, Mike and Amber walked in. Andy's sisters were familiar with all of our visitors, and they were included in our conversation. Before long, it seemed like we branched off into little groups to visit, and Andy's two sisters ended up chatting between themselves.

As the doors opened, my head turned to see the surgeon walking out with an x-ray film in his hand and a very grim look on his face. My heart started racing and I thought for sure he was coming out to tell us Clara was dead. Of everyone sitting there in the waiting room, he came and sat down next to me and started talking. At first, I don't think everyone noticed he was there and I asked him to wait a moment and called them all over. On one hand I felt good that I was the one he came to first, as if he recognized that I was the primary one that cared for Clara. Then on the other hand I wondered what the girls were thinking about that. As everyone quickly gathered around, there was no more time for my thinking, just time to listen. The surgeon said that the surgery went well, and to my surprise I felt a big relief. As much as I would complain at times that it seemed like I would be taking care of Clara for the rest of my life, I still felt relief at this news. The surgeon did tell us that when the anesthesiologist put the breathing tube down her throat that some fluid squirted out. In my mind I was thinking it was good that some of that fluid came out, no matter how it happened. He showed us the x-ray and the reality of this metal rod attached to her bone with screws hit me. I asked if we could see her and he said not just yet, her blood pressure was a bit low, so they were slowly bringing her out of anesthesia. There was a lot of joy on the waiting room, the girls starting calling their husbands and some of Clara's grandchildren to give them the good news.

I now sat there overwhelmingly disappointed. Her surgery was just one hurdle to clear. We still did not know what else was wrong with Clara, why she was so weak, what this mass was in her lungs. I thought of how difficult it was for Clara to get up and down before she had this metal rod in her leg. I kept getting visual images of her laying in a bed in the nursing home, slowly withering away. I felt sick that she survived the surgery, but tried to sit there looking happy. How could I ever express such feelings without sounding like my true concern was about me? I remembered hearing before those residents of nursing homes that have regular visitors usually get far better treatment than those that do not. Since the staff does not know when someone will be checking in they keep the patient in good care constantly. I had already mentally planned on going to the nursing home each day. I wondered if the other ones would be good about stopping in. I thought of how when Clara would be admitted to the hospital in the past, her one daughter would always come after work and stay until visiting hours were over. That was a short termed stay, how would they do with long termed? I was thinking of things in the future and I still had to call my sons and give them an update. When I called Mike and told him all turned out well, he said, "So it looks like Grand mom will eventually come back home, huh?" I said, "Yeap." By my tone he picked up right away I did not consider that good news. As he commented on it, I panicked thinking if he could pick up on it, what about anyone else in the waiting room with us? I quickly changed my tone of voice to an upbeat, positive one for the rest of our conversation. I sat there thinking I was going to vomit, I just felt sick. I knew Clara was in no condition to come home, she needed the rehabilitation at the nursing home, and I knew I was in no condition to care for Clara in this condition. Plus, we were still back to the original problem that led to the broken femur in the first place, that had not yet been diagnosed. What was that unknown mass in her left lung that was noticed when she was first brought to the emergency room? Was Clara slowly dying, and the process was interrupted with this broken leg? Would this just drag out her misery even more? My hope of Clara going to sleep peacefully one night and just never waking up, seemed all but impossible now. How could I take the news that surgery went very well, as devastating news? As I sat there with many thoughts and unpleasant images running through my head, out of the corner of my eye I saw the surgeon re-emerge. He had the same grim look on his face he did when he came out after her surgery. Again, he came and sat down next to me. This time, Andy and the girls quickly gathered around. The doctor began that they were having a difficult time bringing Clara out of anesthesia. Her blood pressure and heart rate were very low. Each time medicine would be administered to bring her pressure and heart rate up she would respond temporarily. The medication only lasted about ten minutes then all of her vitals would drop again. He needed to know if we wanted her kept alive on a machine. I could not believe this news. The girls seemed to have a hard time digesting what was being said. I understood and felt relief for the first time since Clara broke her leg. I thought, what is wrong with you Michele? The girls became understandably hysterical, and Andy tried to comfort them the best he could. Now, I sat with the doctor with him asking me what should be done. I knew Clara had a durable health care document that stated that she did not want to be kept alive on machines if there was no hope of her making a recovery. I did not want the girls to know the doctor was asking me this life or death question about their mother. I also feared that in the emotion of the moment, if the girls had to make a decision like that concerning their own mother, they would say to keep her alive on machines only to later regret it. I told the doctor that Clara had a great love for life and I have seen her fight to stay alive. With that being said, I added that Clara had specifically written her wishes that if she was in a position where there was no hope, she did not want to be kept alive on machines. I asked the doctor if we were to the point that there was no hope and he shook his head yes. I told him her durable health care documents were in her files with her wishes if he needed to confirm what I related. I then asked him if he understood what needed to be done. He said yes. I knew that meant all of the machines were going to be turned off. So I asked if Clara's daughters could come back to say goodbye, he said, "Not now, when it is over." My insides were shaking. The doctor just sat quietly next to me for a minute as I was thinking of how just two days earlier Andy said he was going to step up to the plate as his mother's appointed health care agent. Yet here I am, the only one left in this room to make this actual life or death decision. In my heart, I knew I really was not making any decision; Clara had made her own decision a few years before. I really was trying to take care of Clara, even in this way. Then it hit me, Clara was going to die peacefully in her sleep. She was put under anesthesia, and never woke up. It wasn't exactly like I hoped would happen in her own bed, but the nightmare I imagined of her going to the nursing home was over. I was able to take care of her down to the end, although I hated the broken leg part and the miserable pain that followed, she still died peacefully. As I was deep in my own thoughts, I did not notice at first that the doctor was gone. As I looked up to see where he went, I saw Andy running after him down the hallway. He spoke with the doctor briefly, and then came over to me. He told me he wanted to be sure that the doctor knew what his mother's wishes were. Of course, he had run after his sisters, so he did not know about the conversation I already had with the doctor. It made me feel better that in his mind, he did not want that to fall on me and he was trying to step up to his responsibilities. Now was the waiting for it all to be over. Even though Clara was not declared clinically dead, to me we already received the news that she was dead. It was a foregone conclusion. The girls started making calls explaining how things had taking a turn for the worse. I felt bad for my family and our friends to be with us during such a stressful time, but it was also strengthening having them with us.

It must have been another forty-five minutes before a team of three doctors, including the surgeon emerged to tell us that Clara was dead. The girls seemed shocked by the news, and I was bewildered at their reaction. One of them flipped a chair and screamed towards me and my family, "I bet you are all happy now, you got your wish." With that she stormed out of the waiting room screaming her husband's name, with the other one following. Incredibly, at that moment her husband appeared. He had arrived at the hospital, but due to the late hour, could only enter the hospital through the emergency room for security reasons. He was lost wandering the hallways looking for us, when he heard his wife's voice. I'm sure quite a bit of the hospital heard her voice in her distress. The timing of his arrival was unbelievable, and since Andy had just run after his sisters again, I could point him in her direction. It was obvious he was just what she needed for comfort. I asked the doctors when we could see her and they said they would clean her up, remove the tubes, and then someone would be out to get us. I thanked them for their time and kindness. Then I sat there replaying the outburst towards me and my family. Then I thought, 'I am happy, I did get my wish, but how could she know that?' In my heart, I really do believe my wish that evening was all about Clara, not about me getting a break from caring for Clara. At this point Andy returned, somewhat shaken but in control. He worried for his sisters. I told our visitors that we really appreciated them coming, but we had a long night ahead of us and for them to go home. They all stayed put. Who knows what to do in these situations? In time, the girls and the one husband returned to the waiting room. A nurse appeared saying we could see Clara now. They were still waiting for the other husband to arrive and they seemed conflicted as to what to do. I said I would wait and keep an eye out for him and escort him back to the recovery area. Andy walked back with his sisters. It wasn't long before the other husband arrived, with their teenaged daughter. As we walked back, I saw them all huddled around Clara. Andy's sister grabbed onto her daughter as they grieved together. I went over to Andy to give him a hug and he grabbed onto me and started wailing. I told myself to be strong for him. I think it startled his sisters to hear him crying so loudly. I knew it was in part about seeing them so sad, in part about his mother's passing, and in part because he never wanted to look at his mother dead. As I was walking him out of the recovery area, he said, "I never wanted to look at her dead." Despite that, I knew he walked back there to support his sisters. I wondered if they would ever realize the sacrifice Andy made for them that day. As we returned to the waiting room, my family and our friends surrounded Andy with love and support. I went out into the hallway to call Mike to let him know. Mike is very strong emotionally like me, and the few times he has broken down and cried in the past felt like stabs to my heart. He broke down on the phone but immediately pulled himself together to ask how his Dad was. He was going to drive up. I told him that it was late, by now it was around 11:00 p.m., his Dad was going to want to go home and go to bed. If his Dad knew that he was making the two hour trip up after working a long day, it would just be an added worry on him. With the hospital waiting area being empty other than us, my voice apparently traveled and Andy overheard our conversation. He said, "Please tell Mike not to come tonight." Mike agreed to come the next morning. Moments later a nurse came out and asked to speak with me. She asked me if we had pre-arranged funeral plans, we did not other than the secret obituary I had saved on my computer. The nurse handed me a brochure explaining what documents would be needed to make Clara's funeral arrangements and asked what funeral home we would be using. I told her I would gather the information and give it to her as soon as I could. Why come to me, she had been back in the area with Clara's daughters? In times past, I had tried to feel Clara out on this subject. I remembered once telling her that Andy and I had decided if something happened to us, we would want to be cremated. I asked her if she had any feelings on that matter and she simply replied, "Once I'm dead, what do I care, I won't know what is going on." That was the most I could get from her. I went to Andy and told him that the hospital needed to know what the funeral arrangements were. He said if it was up to him, he prefers cremation, but that whatever his sisters decided he would support. That was the next problem. How do I bring this subject up when they are sitting and mourning with their dead mother? Andy said he could not go back again and see his mother laying their dead. By now, Zack had arrived, and Andy seemed like he was scolding him telling him he didn't have to come. I told Andy that Zack wanted to support him, stop being the parent for the moment and let Zack do just that. Andy truly appreciated it, but felt bad for Zack to drive over by himself on this cold, dark night into such a stressful situation. I asked Andy if it was okay with him, I would go back and try to see what his sisters feelings were on the funeral arrangements. When I did, one of the girls was sitting on the gurney with Clara, the other stroking her head. I wondered if this was a typical difference between men and women. Andy could not stand to be next to his dead mother, the girls could not stand the thought of leaving her side. I asked if I could 'visit' with Clara for a moment and they said, "Sure." I needed my time with her. As I went around the other side of the bed I stroked her face a bit. Her leg was out a bit from under the covers and she had deep, dark bruises on her leg. I wondered if the one bruise on her lower leg was from when her foot got trapped under the weight of her leg when she fell getting out of the shower. There were areas where her skin had broken down during the four day hospital stay. Another wound was obviously from surgery. I wished that when she coded two days before she was never revived. Looking at her purple bruises and incision was sickening. How sad that this poor woman had to go through surgery for nothing, but still felt relieved that her death was peaceful. I was lost in my own thoughts for a few moments, then told the girls that I was sorry to have to bring this up, but the hospital needed to know what funeral arrangements we had in mind. They were very gracious about it, and one had strong feelings about which funeral home she wanted her mother's services held at. I asked if they wanted a plot or a mausoleum and the same one said she did not want her mother buried in the ground. I did not have the courage to even ask if cremation was a consideration, because I felt it would be an offensive question to them. So it was decided which funeral home would be used, and the cemetery was not as specific, as long as they had a mausoleum. I asked if they wanted to be involved in making the arrangements, or if they wanted Andy and me to take care of all the details. They both said they wanted us to make the arrangements. I went over to the nurse to inform her of the decision and she said we needed to call the funeral home and set things up. Thankfully, someone knew what to do! I returned to the waiting area and briefed Andy and he said, "Whatever they want."

I called the funeral home, and the kind gentleman that answered the phone said they would be right over to pick her up. I went back to let the girls know that the funeral home was on their way, and that Andy did not want to see their mother laying there so I was taking him home. They understood, and with that I emerged from the recovery room and we left with our entourage. I had hoped that the girls would leave soon too and get some rest, but was glad we would not be there for the emotion of them leaving. I offered for Andy to ride home with Zack, but he said he would stay with me. I like that Andy can draw strength from me during difficult times. On the way home he said he felt it was all for the best, that he too wondered if his mother was dying and knew her stay in a nursing home, would not be good. He said he never wanted the last image of his mother to be of her dead, but he did not want his sisters to face her without him. I told him he could work hard to replace that image with a happier one, especially since the prior four days had lots of unpleasant images we needed to block out.

Chapter Eight

THE DAYS OF THE FUNERAL

We went to bed, but it wasn't long before I was up gathering the documents the hospital brochure said we would need. Andy was up early the next morning, and while he was in the shower, I was on the phone calling around to different cemeteries to find out which ones had mausoleums. Since Clara only had $1500 in life insurance and about $3500 in the bank, it was quickly becoming obvious we were far short of what we needed. I was shocked to learn that a burial in the ground cost less than being put in a mausoleum. I called the funeral home to make an appointment to come in that morning to finalize arrangements and made another appointment at the cemetery where my father was buried. When at the funeral home, I expressed my shock at the cost involved at the cemetery. The funeral director actually had the nerve to talk negatively about how the cemetery takes advantage of people during these difficult times. I looked at the paperwork the funeral director just provided, at the list of charges from embalming, to various charges for using the funeral home, I had to bite my tongue because he offered no bargain himself. When we got out to the car, Andy thanked me for keeping my mouth shut when the funeral director made his negative comment. I laughed that he knew me so well. The cost of the funeral home already exceeding any monies Clara had and we knew the rest was coming out of our pocket. Through the years, money always seemed to be a dividing factor somehow. Once Clara sold her modest house and moved in to live with us, whenever we would make a major purchase, Clara would tell me that one or both of the girls would express concern that we were using her funds for our purchases. Andy was a hard worker with a good paying job so I could never understand the accusations. I remember one time asking Andy if we should show them our prior years tax return so that they could see that we can afford the things we buy and he basically asked me if I was nuts, it was none of their business. He said as long as they went to their mother saying stuff, he considered it gossip. If they were really that concerned, they could come to him and he would address it then. It always bothered me. Even when Andy bought me a beautiful blue diamond ring for our 25th wedding anniversary, I did not tell Clara for months. I knew she would be excited for me, and naturally share the news with her girls, and then the money complaints would resurface. I wondered at times how they thought we could buy so many things and take so many vacations on the amount of money Clara gained from the sale of her house. When Clara first starting going to the doctors, she needed so many medications to address untreated long term problems, her medications were quite expensive. Clara's savings dwindled down for a number of reasons, none of which was for our financial gain. When Clara would relate something that one of her girls said about her money, I would ask her if she was concerned that we were mismanaging her money. She always said she was not worried at all. Eventually, when someone commented to her about my beautiful ring in her presence, she was upset that I never told her about it, (with her limited vision, she never noticed it). I told her that I knew she would tell her girls and I didn't want her to have to hear again that we were using her apparent endless supply of money. Clara said, "Do you know how sick I am of hearing about that money? Sometimes I wished I never got any." I knew how irritating it was to me to have these ongoing accusations made, but I never stopped to think how hurtful it was for Clara to hear these things as a parent. It had to be hard for Clara to hear her daughters accuse her son, that she was living with, of stealing from her and not having her best interests at heart. Of course, I don't think they ever thought Andy was stealing from her, but that I was. Clara told me once that it probably relieved their conscience that I did so much for her, for them to think my motive was for financial gain. When Clara said that, I asked her point blank if that is what she thought and she said, "Michele, I know you take care of me because of how much you love me." Clara wasn't sentimental in her expressions, so when she would make a statement like that, it would mean a lot to me. So now we are heading up to the cemetery, we have already added $1000 of our own money to Clara's proceeds to settle the funeral home expenses. Obviously, the cemetery expenses would be all out of our pocket. I about fell off of my chair to find out the cemetery cost would be close to $5000! How could a one day viewing at a funeral home and a slot in a mausoleum cost over $10,000.00? What a rip off. I went into business mode at the cemetery and started questioning the validity of some of the charges itemized. The cost of digging a grave, placing the casket, and filling the grave in, was less than the cost of sliding her casket in what amounted to me as a drawer in the mausoleum. The salesman, oops I mean director tried to come up with an explanation, but then Andy interrupted and said, "Basically, it is what it is." The director agreed. I realized that was my cue to shut up. I'm trying to negotiate a reasonable price to honor his sister's wishes, but forgot to be sensitive of Andy's feelings. This was not a business deal, but his mother's final arrangements. When we left I apologized for how I handled things. Andy laughed and said that I turned into quite the business woman in there, but he could see that it was futile, the price was non-negotiable. I apologized again for not being more sensitive to his pain, and he said that it was not a problem. He knew then he had the advantage and said, "Can we go to the Lazy Boy store and look for new chairs?" For months he had been saying he wanted new chairs for our family room, and I told him there was nothing wrong with the chairs we had. I told him he was taking advantage of the situation and he said he just wanted to do something non hospital or non funeral related. How could I argue with that? I thought it strange that we left the cemetery to go shopping, but then I thought, well really, what really is the right thing to do? When we got home, Mike and Tanya had arrived and it was comforting for us all to be together. Andy called his sisters to let them know the arrangements. I talked with them telling them I wanted to get a collage of photos together to display at the funeral, if that was alright with them. They agreed and later called and said they had some pictures they would drop off so I could copy them and use them also. It felt like the division was back, us and them. I continued to wonder if they blamed me for their mother's death, since she fell on my watch. I was at the craft store buying a large frame for the collage, when they dropped off the photos at the house. There were more than I anticipated, and with what I had, I needed a second frame. It was therapeutic for me to do this. Once I finished it was time to get the funeral programs together. I wanted to do them myself; because I wanted to be sure Clara had nice programs at her funeral. How do you sum up over eighty years of life in two pages? I felt satisfied with the dignity of how Clara's funeral program came out. Before Clara's health really declined, we had a photographer come to our house for some family photos. Clara was in some of them, and the photographer snapped a few of Clara by herself. There was a perfect photo for the front.

We arrived at the funeral home early so I could set up the two collages I put together and set out the programs. To my surprise the rest of Andy's family was already there waiting for the funeral director to finish the last details before the viewing. I went upstairs to set my things up. I felt a bit nervous, but I was glad when I saw Clara lying in the casket looking peaceful. They did not cake on the makeup as I have seen done before, and she really just looked like she was taking a nap. Then an eerie feeling came over me and I rushed back downstairs to join the family and wait for permission for the official viewing to begin.

The day of Clara's viewing was Super bowl Sunday. We had lots of support during the afternoon viewing, but a bit less in the evening once the game started. Even Zack and Mike asked they could go home to watch the game. For some that may have seemed disrespectful, but to me funerals are for the living. If that was not helping them mourn their grandmother's passing, I was not going to insist that they stay. Alice, Clara's old aide that had become her good friend was sitting out in the hallway. I went over to her as she was quite distraught. She expressed that she felt like Clara knew she was going to die. She said in December when she had come by for a visit, Clara asked her to get out her jewelry and take whatever she wanted. Clara only had costume jewelry, and Alice was not a big jewelry wearer. Alice felt like Clara wanted her to have something to remember her by. I was shocked to hear this but made me realize when I wondered if Clara was in the process of dying, she was wondering the same thing about herself.

In the evening, one of Clara's granddaughter's came over and sat down next to me. She thanked me for the care I had given her grandmother for so many years. I was appreciative to hear those words; I told her I was fretting wondering if they held me responsible for her death. She assured me she did not. Some time later, one of Clara's daughters came over to me and asked to see me privately. The tone of her voice made me feel like there was going to be some sort of confrontation. I was completely wrong. She told me that it had come to her attention that I was concerned that they blamed me for their mother's death. She firmly assured me that was not the case. They knew that I had done my best. I apologized that Clara fell on my watch. It felt like that part of things was settled. The next day was the funeral, it was very well supported. I went into the room to set up my funeral programs and found Maria, Clara's last aide sitting outside in the hallway. She told me that she felt Clara knew she was going to die. I asked her why she said that. Maria said that for a couple of weeks before Clara's fall, when Maria would be ready to leave Clara would say, "Maria, give me a hug, you never know, I might not be here the next time you come." This was comforting yet torturous information for me to hear. The fact that Clara died under anesthesia continued to comfort me. The thought of Clara agonizing about her own death, made me feel so sad for her. I could not help but wonder how many hours she sat there by herself scared, or when she was helped to bed if she worried she might never wake up. I decided to concentrate on the positive aspect of things, that Clara did not suffer long term.

My brother Jim actually delivered the funeral talk and was able to include some of his own personal experiences that he had in visiting Clara in the past, and during her last hospital stay. During the funeral talk, at times it looked like Clara was breathing, her chest rising up and down. I had to convince myself that my eyes were playing tricks on me. The talk was finished, and the funeral director instructed the family members to pay their last respects. As Andy walked out, he burst into tears and cried loudly. Of course I was at his side trying to support him. A co-worker of his was standing in the hallway, and he stepped toward Andy to hug him and Andy embraced him tightly. It was sad to see him so broken. What was going through my mind? I was wondering if I looked heartless because I was not crying. I was trying to think what was expected or acceptable behavior from me. Should I cry too? Would that help Andy or make it about me needing comfort from him? As we walked down the steps to the family vehicle arranged by the funeral home, the pressure was over. Once out of the funeral home and into the vehicle, Clara's children were pulling themselves together. It was nice sitting there so we could observe all of our friends as they were coming out of the funeral home, some of which we did not notice while inside. After the cemetery, we went back to my mother's house for a meal. As the day came to a close, one of Clara's daughter's hugged me and thanked me for everything. I was not sure if that was everything related to the funeral or everything related to the care I provided. At that point, it was the first thank you I had ever received from her, so I decided to take it as a thank you for everything.

Chapter Nine

LIFE AFTER CLARA

All the times I had thought how much easier life would be once Clara was gone, but I never went beyond that thought. What would I do once she was gone? I did not realize how difficult the transition would be. One of the most surprising side effects of Clara's death was the recurring dreams I would have. They were actually nightmares, because each dream would be about Clara falling and me trying to get her help. When I would tell some of my friends about my recurring nightmares I would always be told the same thing, 'You have no reason to feel guilty, you took excellent care of Clara.' I don't think guilt was the problem. It wasn't about the blame game. The day Clara fell getting out of the shower, I felt was a combination of bad circumstances and honestly, the responsibility fell on her. Once she made up her mind she was falling, despite my pleas not to, and released her body weight, she became like dead weight. Even though Andy and Zack were home and are quite strong, I don't think they would have even been able to hold her up if they were in my position. For me I think it was more about all the things I had done, all the sacrifices I had made, all the times I injured my own body in my effort to help Clara-all seemed to be defined by the end. Clara fell on my watch, plain and simple. I don't believe it was guilt, but sheer disappointment at my defeat at the end. There was also overwhelming aggravation and anger at Clara's doctor for ignoring my concerns the weeks prior to her death. I felt the care I was trying to get her was blocked by the very person that was supposed to provide it. No matter what the cause, the dreams were there, every night. For almost two months I had a different dream but the theme was the same, Clara fell and I was urgently trying to get her help. Once I would wake up from my dream, usually after about three hours of sleep, I was too anxious to fall back to sleep. In part I did not want to take a chance of the dream continuing. It would be crazy dreams sometimes based on actual events that had happened. One night I dreamed about helping Clara down the steps of a friend's house we were visiting. Many years before, I had helped Clara down the steps of this friend's house, without incident. In my dream however, Clara fell down the final step. For some reason my car was not available or would not work. I placed her on a dolly, the kind that I've seen people use to stack up boxes on to transport. Dreams are not based on logic; at least mine never are, so for some reason I had a dolly available. I strapped Clara to this dolly; she is standing upright with bungee cords holding her on. I am behind her trying to run her home to our house. For several miles I was successful in keeping a fast pace then the wheels would fall off of the dolly. I stood there with complete anxiety wondering how I was going to get Clara the help she needed. I would wake up and my heart would be pounding. I'm not so dense that I could not see the correlation. The night Clara fell getting out of the shower, I was so close to successfully getting her out of the shower, and when I felt we were just about in home stretch, the fall. Then there was the frantic cry for help, then Andy being put on hold with 911, then the hospital being backed up. I would lie in bed logically trying to reason things out, but I was still too scared to go back to sleep. One night, I talked to a very good friend of mine, who had become a caregiver at the end of his wife's battle with leukemia. He understood the dreams, the feeling of panic that you forgot to do something important, he said for me to give it time, it would resolve. After almost sixty days of this, I needed sleep. I went to my primary physician and explained my dilemma. She prescribed a sleep aid for ten days to break the vicious cycle I was in. I was so looking forward to getting peaceful sleep. The first night I took the sleep aid I did not have any dreams, none that I remember anyway. I slept for five hours, a bit short of the eight hours I thought I would get, but still far better than the three I had been getting. For ten straight days I would sleep dream free, but only for five hours. The first night off the medication I could not sleep at all. I called for another round. After really reading the information flier that came with the sleep aid, it explained that once you went off the medicine, you may experience insomnia for a couple of nights. I figured I was just postponing the inevitable so decided not to take anymore. The good news was the dreams did not return. The bad news was I was back to getting about three hours of sleep a night. Within days I was starting to get a bit more sleep, but have not slept a complete night since.

Another 'side effect' of Clara's death was what amounted to panic attacks. One day I was in a department store and had walked to the register to pay for my purchases and there were a couple of customers in line in front of me. Without warning or cause, my heart started pounding, I broke out in a sweat and I felt like I had to flee the store, as if I had to be somewhere urgent. At first I was startled and confused by what was going on. I checked my watch; it was the time I used to have to be at dialysis to pick Clara up. I was panicking as if I forgot to take care of Clara. As I continued standing in line, I had to have an internal talk with myself reminding myself I did not have to leave to get Clara; that assignment was over. When it was my turn to pay for my items, my heart had settled back into a normal rhythm, but I felt nervous, like when you have too much caffeine. I actually experienced this several more times on other occasions, but I knew then to check the time first. Sure enough, each time it happened was when I normally would have been taking Clara to or from dialysis. My body and internal clock was still programmed to Clara time. My friend was right, in time these things resolved themselves.

I reflect back on that conversation I had, well that spat I had with Clara's daughter after returning from the cruise. I wondered if through the years I had alienated them, by them having the impression that I was a one woman show with Clara's care. Then again, the reality was, I did do the majority. I knew of others that never got any family help, so I was always happy for the break that would come on Wednesday and Saturday. Upon reflection I decided that was more of an excuse on her part not to have to recognize that I truly was her mother's caregiver. That's just my opinion of course. I also think back to that fateful night that Clara broke her leg and when her daughter showed up and said, "Why didn't you call me? I would have come over and helped you." I remembered feeling incredulous that she would make such a statement. I've wondered about all those times when they knew I was sick and did nothing additional to help with their mother. Was all that was needed was for me to call them and ask for help? Clara often hated to ask her own children for things that she thought would be an inconvenience to them, which I never could understand. Was it possible at times they may have even offered to help but Clara told them not to worry about it? I often used discernment in anticipating and filling Clara's needs, so that was the expectation I had for her daughters when I was sick. Could I have saved myself years of frustration and resentment by just calling them directly and asking for help when I was sick or following surgery? I don't think so, but I don't know. I never really tried it to know if it would have worked or not. Hopefully, I will remember if ever in a caregiver's position again, to have better communication skills with other family members as to my expectations or requests for help.

I find myself much more in tune to senior citizens now. One small example of this was recently when my husband and I were on a trip, taking a tour, and there was a retired woman in our tour group traveling alone. At our first stop, we were told we could look around and to meet back in fifteen minutes at the tour bus. I could detect nervousness on this woman's part and I asked her if she was okay. She said she doesn't have a good sense of direction, and she was afraid if she looked around, she would not find her way back to the tour bus. So she was just going to stand by the tour bus until it was time to move to the next location. Andy and I took her under our wing, each stop she would stick to us like glue. We both felt good that this woman that we just met felt comfortable with us, and she ended up being enjoyable company. Even though at times I feel like a senior citizen magnet, there is a feeling of satisfaction in helping other people.

I have another friend that is in her seventies, and due to the poor health of her and her husband, they sometimes need help with transportation to doctor's appointments. The eye doctor they see every three months is the same one Clara had, so it is enjoyable seeing the staff again when I take them.

I know my circumstances were great compared to many others. Often friends or family members would praise me for the quality of care I provided for Clara and the difficulties that came along with her care. I would often comment on the women that have to work full time jobs and then come home to an aged parent that needs their help. My amazement is with the ones that care for both aged parents, especially if one has Alzheimer's. I have a friend that is going through her second bout with cancer, and out of three other siblings, she provides ninety-five percent of the care her aged mother needs.

All and all, I feel like being a caregiver made me a better person. Even when I would think dark thoughts, I recognize it was merely the stress of a sometimes difficult situation.

For a long time I didn't really miss Clara, because thoughts of Clara were always associated with her needs due to her conditions or diseases. It's been about two years now since she has died, and sometimes I just think of me and Clara chatting, laughing, discussing life. I can now think about her without the crappy part of it always being associated. Clara was a pleasant old soul in a lot of ways. Clara did not have an easy life from the time her mother died when she was just starting out as a teenager; to the idiot she married and abandoned her and their children. She was not a bitter person at all. I think my life is better for knowing her, and I think her life was better for knowing me. That is an incredible gift, to know that I actually improved the quality of someone else's life!

So I feel like I'm part of a very special group, that of caregiver's. At times when folks ask me, "What do you do?" the first thing that comes to my mind is to say, "I'm a caregiver." Then I have to remind myself that statement is no longer true, although I believe I will always be one in my heart. I have been able to help a few others when they have experienced the loss of a parent that they have cared for. There are so many conflicting emotions, and to actually feel relief at their death can make you feel like a terrible human being. Knowing that someone else has had feelings similar to their own, has often been a comfort. My hope is by writing this book it may help family members that are not the primary caregivers to give more thought to help the person that is. For the ones that are primary caregivers, and at times wish their aged parent dead, not to feel like they are a dreadful member of society. Whenever possible, try to use humor to help you through the difficult times. If you ever find yourself in a position of washing your aged parent after they have soiled themselves, please remember, and keep the washcloth out of their reach!!!

Are you a born caregiver? Is there such a thing? How does it change you?

This not just for caregivers a caregiver exposé.
Help others to understand & also esp as they could end up being a caregiver themselves.

19545033R00061

Made in the USA
Charleston, SC
30 May 2013